Handbook for Pediatric Health Problems at Home and on the Road

Handbook for Pediatric Health Problems at Home and on the Road

Dr. Christopher S. Ryder

MB, BCh. D.C.H. (London)

F.C.P. (S.A.) F.A.A.P.

LCCN 2004093260

ISBN 0-9755260-2-2

Dedication

This book is dedicated to my best friend and wife, Alixe, and to my son, David. Thank you for all your love, patience, support, and understanding.

Table of Contents

Foreword

B.K. VARMA, M.D.

As the world becomes more accessible in our age of internet, cruise ships, jets, and cars, more families are traveling with children. But the joy of a vacation may be ruined by faulty planning, lack of knowledge of the destination, visa requirements,, endemic disease, and cultural differences.

Christopher Ryder MD, an outstanding pediatrician and a parent with a young son, has traveled extensively. He has personally experienced the joys and trials of traveling with his family and he describes these "encounters of travel kind" in this book.

The book succeeds admirably, providing state of the art information in a comprehensive and easy to understand manner. It deals with planning, preparation for travel, and prevention and treatment of common illnesses and accidents experienced by traveling families. Travel related medical and non medical problems are discussed.

Although Dr. Ryder originally intended this book just for travelers it will be an invaluable resource for expectant parents, parents planning a foreign adoption and for all families with children.

As a professional colleague, I highly recommend this all encompassing book for families both at home and on the road, medical personnel and travel clinics.

B.K. Varma, M.D.
Chairman Department of Pediatrics
Pinnacle Health Hospital, Harrisburg, Pennsylvania
Clinical Professor of Pediatrics, Penn. State University of Medicine, Hershey, Pennsylvania

Foreword

BORIS SKURKOVICH, M.D.

If you have children, you need this book! Comprehensive and easy to use, it will inform, empower, and encourage you. The author of this book, Dr. Christopher Ryder, is one of the best pediatricians that I have ever known with more than 25 years of experience caring for children and their families. His incredible depth and breadth of knowledge allowed him to write this most comprehensive, well researched and practical book. It should be used not only during travel with children, but in every day life as well.

The medical kit that accompanies this book is so well thought through that I could not come up with any suggestions about how to improve it. If you have this book and the kit you can feel very comfortable that you are prepared to face any potential medical issue that may face your child.

Boris Skurkovich, M.D.
Clinical Associate Professor of Pediatrics
Brown Medical School

Director, International Adoption Clinic
Hasbro Children's Hospital
Providence, Rhode Island

Introduction

SOON AFTER COMPLETING MY MEDICAL TRAINING, I left South Africa and visited England for the first time. The sense of freedom and independence I felt was exhilarating. I remember it as though it were yesterday the excitement I felt as I explored London. I would rise early and jog along the often damp pavements, marveling at the sights and sounds of that great city as it woke to greet a new day.

Europe followed England, and even after I returned to South Africa, the generous vacations I enjoyed enabled me to continue to travel. I then went to the Middle East and worked in Bahrain for three years before settling in the United States.

Now those month long annual vacations are but a dream, but my wife and I still use our free time to indulge ourselves and to share with our son the adventures that travel offers. Together we have traveled through much of Europe, parts of Africa, Asia, and America.

Some years ago, friends of ours were taking their six-year-old to China for three months and asked us what they should take with them so they would be prepared to treat minor illnesses while away. We suggested they buy a first aid kit. They arrived on our doorstep, bulging shopping bags in hand, and together we unpacked a variety of drug store first aid and medical kits on our dining room table. As we checked the contents of each one it became obvious that most of them contained not much more than a collection of band aids and bandages and medications suitable only for adults. Not one of these kits was suitable for a family traveling with a child. In fact, none of the medications contained in any of these kits could even be swallowed by a young child! Traveling with children requires a different sort of preparation and this was the inspiration for the creation of a child-friendly travel kit.

My wife and I then started to assemble some basic items that we knew we would use when traveling with our child. As the kit evolved it became obvious that this was something that every family could use both at home and while on vacation. Many families rely on their pediatrician or family doctor for advice when faced with the common ailments of childhood. However, when they are away from home this is not always possible, so I felt it necessary to write a book to accompany the kit. This book covers many of the more common accidents and illnesses that a parent might encounter both while at home and while traveling.

This book is divided into five sections:

A) **A pediatric medical kit.** This section discusses what to include in a pediatric medical kit.

B) **Traveling with children.** This covers the preparation for travel in the United States and abroad. It includes discussion of common problems such as earaches while flying, jetlag, and motion sickness, as well as less common and more serious diseases such as malaria and altitude sickness. It also includes a section on traveling with children who have chronic diseases such as asthma and diabetes. As a pediatrician, part of my job involves taking care of children adopted from foreign countries so I have included a chapter on bringing home the foreign adoptee.

C) **Common childhood illnesses and their symptoms.** This includes most of the common sicknesses that children get as they grow up such as fevers, coughs and colds, strep throat, constipation, vomiting, and diarrhea.

D) Common summer ailments. The most important topic covered here is the prevention of sunburn.

E) Accident prevention, injuries and emergencies. Even though this book discusses exotic diseases such as malaria, the most likely reason your child will land in the hospital while traveling in the United States or abroad is an accident. **Motor vehicle accidents are the leading cause of death while traveling.** Accidents are also one of the most common causes of death in childhood in the United States! This section includes the prevention of some of the more common accidents as well as prevention of extremely rare events such as lightening strikes.

Some of the sections go into extensive detail on how to manage specific problems. This applies particularly to the sections on traveler's diarrhea, diarrhea and dehydration, and fevers. These are very common problems during childhood and while traveling. While most families who use this kit and book will have ready access to medical care, others may be in a remote location and will have to cope with these problems entirely on their own. It is my hope that this book contains sufficient information to get these families through these illnesses.

This book does not contain an exhaustive list of all the problems your children are likely to develop, just the common ones. References are given for more detailed information and further reading for parents. The parents' stress level will be higher away from home and away from familiar surroundings and familiar and trusted health care.

• Parents should use common sense and parental intuition.

- If in doubt, seek experienced medical help. Guidelines are given for when to seek expert medical help and how to locate physicians abroad, including physicians who speak English.

Note: **This book is not intended to replace your child's doctor or to replace medical advice and treatment while away.**

The accompanying pediatric travel kit does not contain all the medications your child may need. The medications enclosed are just starting doses and, like all medications, have expiration dates. These medications will have to be replaced from time to time. Suggestions are made for additional items and medications that you may like to include in your child's medical kit. Guidelines on dosing and how to use these medications are included in this book.

Your medical kit may not contain any prescription medications such as antibiotics. These have to be obtained from a physician. If you intend to travel outside the United States, especially to developing countries, you should discuss with your child's physician other medications you should take with you. Any chronic or routine medications that your child is taking should, obviously, also be included.

Despite all the warnings contained in this book, traveling abroad should be fun and educational. Understanding and learning the reasons for various precautions will help you and your children follow them. The more prepared you are, the less likely you are to need this medical kit or to need medical care in a foreign country.

~

1

A Children's
Medical Kit

This chapter discusses the items suitable for a medical kit for children. You may have purchased this book as part of a children's first-aid/travel kit. Your pediatric medical kit should contain many of the essential items and medications that you will need to have at home and while traveling. **You will need to purchase other items to complete the kit.** The contents of your kit will vary with the ages of your children and your destination and type of travel.

This chapter goes into extensive detail on the suggested components of a comprehensive medical kit you may want to assemble for prolonged travel to lesser-developed countries. However, most families will only require a more basic medical kit for use at home or for travel in the United States. Below are the recommended contents for such a basic kit for infants and young children.

This chapter also includes suggestions for additional items and medications that you might like to take with you when traveling. There may be essential items you will need to get through a physician if you are traveling to countries where more exotic diseases, such as malaria, may be present. Please discuss this with your child's physician **several weeks before** you are due to depart. When traveling, do not forget to take **your child's routine medications** along, for example, allergy and asthma medications.

All medications have an expiration date. Check the medications in your kit and replace and update them as necessary. This check should take place routinely before any trip and periodically between trips. This will ensure that you always have unexpired medications to use in the event of an emergency. Just as it is a good idea to change the smoke alarm batteries in your house when you adjust your clocks for daylight saving in the spring and fall, it would also be a good time to check your medical kit. As your child grows you may also need to change the formulation of the different medicines, for example *Tylenol* syrup instead of *Tylenol* drops.

All the medications in your medical kit are over-the-counter medications and most can be purchased from your local drugstore. You may have difficulty finding these medications outside the United States, especially in developing countries. Additionally, many medications in developing countries do not have expiration dates printed on their containers. Moreover, many of these medications may have different names outside the United States, for example, paracetamol instead of acetaminophen (*Tylenol*). For all these reasons, it is suggested that you **go through your kit prior to travel and replenish it.**

For further details on how to use these medications, consult the appropriate sections in this book.

Basic Medical Kit for Infants and Young Children

- **Pain and fever medication.**
  1. Acetaminophen (for example, *Tylenol* drops **and** acetaminophen suppositories, either *Feverall* or *Acephen*)
  2. Ibuprofen (for example, *Advil* children's suspension)

- **Allergy, cough and cold medication.**
  1. Saline nose drops
  2. Diphenhydramine (*Benadryl* liquid, *Benadryl* chewable tablets, or *Benadryl* Fastmelt tablets)

- **Medication for "tummy upsets," constipation, diarrhea, and stomachache.**
  1. Electrolyte salts such as *Liquilyte* solution or *Kaoelectrolyte* powder
  2. Glycerine infant suppositories, Milk of Magnesia

- **Ointments and creams.**
  1. Barrier cream or ointment for diaper rashes (*Desitin, A and D Ointment,* or *Triple Paste*)
  2. 1% Hydrocortisone cream or ointment (for example, *Cortaid*)
  3. Antifungal cream to treat yeast diaper rashes (for example, clotrimazole cream, *Lotrimin*)
  4. Anti-bacterial cream for cuts and scrapes (for example, *Triple antibiotic, Neosporin,* or *Bactroban* cream)
  5. Aloe vera gel for burns

- **Basic wound care supplies.** This should include *Band-aids,* gauze swabs, a roll of adhesive tape, an *Ace* bandage, and an antiseptic cleaning solution.

- **Hygiene aids.** This should include an alcohol-based hand sanitizer gel or towelettes such as *Purelle.*

- **Instruments and supplies.**
  1. Flexible digital thermometer
  2. Pair of scissors
  3. 5 ml medication dropper
  4. Disposable gloves
  5. Tweezers to remove splinters and ticks

- **Sunscreen**

- **Insect repellent**

For correct dosage and how to use the medications and supplies, refer to the appropriate sections in this chapter and the relevant sections later in this book.

Medications.

- **Most children's medications are dosed according to weight. It is advisable to know your child's approximate weight so that you can calculate the correct dose of a medication.**

- It is easier to carry tablets than liquids when you travel, but your child should be able to chew or swallow these. Many medications are marketed as pleasant-tasting chewable tablets that are suitable for children as young as two years of age.

- **Keep your kit and all medications in a safe place.**

Pain and fever medication
(Refer also to the section on fever in childhood).

1. **Acetaminophen** (known as paracetamol in many countries)—This is the best known medication used to control fever and mild to moderate pain in children. It is sold in different forms (infant drops, children's elixir or syrup, chewable tablets, tablets, and suppositories) and marketed under a variety of trade names, the most recognized one in the United States being *Tylenol*.

   - **Acetaminophen infant drops** (trade name: *Tylenol* infant drops)—Ideal for treating fever and pain in the first year of life but may also be used in older children. Consult a physician before using in the first two to three months of life. **Any fever or illness in the first two to three months of life should be discussed with a physician.**

      Dosing—the bottle contains a dropper with two marks—at 0.4 ml. (half a dropper) and at 0.8 ml. (full dropper). There are 80 mg. of acetaminophen in 0.8 ml. **Use only the dropper supplied with the bottle.** Not all medication droppers are the same size!

- **Acetaminophen elixir, syrup, suspension liquid—** contains 160 mg. of acetaminophen per 5 ml. (1 tsp.). This is suitable for older infants and pre-school children. It is a less concentrated form than the infant drops.

- **Acetaminophen chewable tablets—**pleasant-tasting tablets which come in two strengths—80 mg. and 160 mg. Chewable tablets are ideal for children two years and older and are easier to carry and administer than the liquid.

- **Acetaminophen tablets and caplets—**These come in a variety of strengths (80 mg. to 500 mg.) and are suitable for adults and older children who can swallow tablets.

- **Acetaminophen suppositories** (trade names: *Feverall* and *Acephen*)—These are inserted rectally and come in a variety of strengths from 80 to 600 mg. For easy administration, coat with *Vaseline* or *KY* jelly before insertion. Hold your child's buttocks together for one to two minutes after inserting the suppository.

    The suppository will melt and be rapidly absorbed. If the suppository has been kept in a warm environment, it may have softened. Place in the refrigerator to firm. A solid suppository is easier to insert!

    Occasionally your child may eject the suppository. Reinsert and hold your child's buttocks together.

ACETAMINOPHEN DOSING CHART

Child's Weight	Infant Drops	Children's Syrup	80 mg Chew tabs	120 mg Suppository
6–8 lbs	0.4 ml	—	—	—
9–11 lbs	0.6 ml	—	—	½
12–18 lbs	0.8 ml	—	—	¾
19–24 lbs	1.2 ml	¾ tsp	1½	1
25–29 lbs	1.6 ml	1 tsp	2	1¼–1½
30–35 lbs	2.0 ml	1¼ tsp	2	1½–2
36–48 lbs	—	1½ tsp	3	2
49–64 lbs	—	2 tsp	4	2½
65–70 lbs.	—	2½ tsp	5	3
71–80 lbs	—	3 tsp	6	4

Note of Caution:

- Do not use in the first two to three months of life without consulting a physician.
- Can be given every four hours, but do not exceed five doses per twenty-four hours.
- Not all teaspoons are equivalent to 5 ml. Use the medicine dropper supplied with the infant drops when using the infant drops. When using the suspension, use the measuring cup supplied with the suspension or the large medicine dropper supplied in the medical kit.
- **Beware!** Some cold medications contain acetaminophen. **Always check the ingredients of other medications you are administering to your child** so that you do not give too large a dose of acetaminophen.
- Acetaminophen is extremely safe when used correctly, but if overdosed, or used for prolonged periods at usual doses, can cause severe liver damage and even be fatal!
- Do not use for longer than three to four days without consulting a physician. Consult a physician earlier if you feel your child's condition is deteriorating. See section titled "Fevers in Children" in this book.
- Acetaminophen is dosed according to body weight. The recommended dose is approximately 4 mg. to 7 mg. per lb. body weight. THE DOSES LISTED HERE ARE THE *MAXIMUM* DOSE and may differ from the recommended dose on the medicine box or bottle.

2. Ibuprofen—Ibuprofen is also extremely effective in treating fever and pain in children and adults. It has the advantage over acetaminophen that the fever-reducing and pain-relieving effects last six to eight hours. It also has an anti-inflammatory effect. Its main disadvantage is that it may cause stomach irritation and bleeding problems. It is extremely safe if used correctly. Ibuprofen is not recommended for infants under six-months of age.
Ibuprofen comes in a variety of forms:

- **Ibuprofen infant concentrated drops** (50 mg./ 1.25 ml.)—This is a concentrated form of ibuprofen and comes with a dropper or syringe. *Note:* **These drops should *not* be administered with a teaspoon or larger medicine dropper.**

- **Ibuprofen Children's Suspension** (100 mg./5 ml.)—This is ideal for older infants and young children. It comes in a pleasant-tasting liquid and is usually very easy to administer. The two best known ibuprofen suspensions are *Motrin Children's Suspension* and *Advil Children's Suspension*.

- **Ibuprofen Chewable Tablets**—These come as 50 mg. and 100 mg. chewable tablets. Both the *Advil* and the *Motrin* brands are pleasant tasting.

- **Ibuprofen Tablets** (200 mg. of ibuprofen per tablet)—These are suitable for adults and older children who can swallow tablets.

IBUPROFEN DOSING CHART

Child's Weight	Infant Drops	Children's Syrup	100 mg. Chewable Tablets
12–16 lbs	1.25 ml	½ tsp	—
17–21 lbs	1.87 ml	¾ tsp	—
22–32 lbs	2.5 ml	1 tsp	1
33–43 lbs	—	1½ tsp	1½
44–65 lbs	—	2 tsp	2
66–80 lbs	—	3 tsp	3

Note of Caution:

- Not recommended for infants below six months of age.
- Give every six to eight hours but not more than three doses in twenty-four hours.
- Do not use for longer than three to four days without consulting a physician.
- If your child's condition is deteriorating, consult a physician.
- Ibuprofen can cause severe gastric irritation, bleeding, and kidney and liver damage. As with all other medications, it is essential to dose accurately.

Additional notes on the use of acetaminophen and ibuprofen:

▶ Neither of these medications will be effective in reducing fever if the child is too warmly clothed or is in a very warm environment.

▶ Neither medication may return your child's temperature to normal but will often lower the temperature by only two or three degrees.

▶ As mentioned in this book in the "Fever" section, the height of your child's fever is less important than how your child is acting.

► Despite the fact that both of these are over the counter medications, both may be extremely toxic if overdosed or if used for too long a period. Always check other medications you are administering to your child to make sure that they do not contain these ingredients.

► If in any doubt, consult a physician.

► Keep these and all other medications out of the reach of children.

Allergy/cough and cold medication

1. **Diphenhydramine allergy liquid and chewable tablets** Diphenhydramine is a very effective medication for allergies and is often marketed under the trade name *Benadryl*. It comes in many forms:

- *Benadryl* Allergy Liquid (12.5 mg./5 ml.).
- *Benadryl* Allergy Chewable Tablets (12.5 mg. per tablet).
- *Benadryl* Allergy Fastmelt Tablets (12.5 mg. per tablet).

suitable for younger children

- *Benadryl* Allergy tablets (25 mg per tablet)—suitable for older children who can swallow tablets.

This medication is very effective for treating the itch associated with hives, insect stings, food allergies, and many other allergic reactions. Diphenhydramine also has a beneficial effect on coughs and the runny nose and sneezing associated with the common cold. For dosing, see the table below.

DIPHENHYDRAMINE (*BENADRYL*) DOSING TABLE

Approximate Weight	Age	Liquid	*Benadryl* allergy chewable tablet or *Benadryl* allergy Fastmelt tablet (12.5 mg)	Tablets (25 mg)
12–20 lbs	6–12 mos	¼–½ tsp	—	
21–26 lbs	12–24 mos	½–1 tsp	½–1	—
27–36 lbs	2–4 yrs	1–1¼ tsp	1—	
37–44 lbs	4–6 yrs	1¼–1½ tsp	1–1½	—
45–90 lbs	6–12 yrs	1½–2 tsp	1½–2	1
>90 lbs	>12 yrs	2–4 tsp	2–4	1–2

- Dosed every 6 hours.
- Usual dose: 0.5 mg per lb. body weight every 6 hours.

Note of Caution:

- Not recommended for infants less than 6 months of age.
- **Benadryl tends to cause drowsiness and should not be taken by adolescents and adults who intend to drive a motor vehicle or operate machinery.**
- Occasionally, *Benadryl* may cause excitability, difficulty falling asleep, and extreme irritability.
- Do **not** use with any other product containing diphenhydramine.
- **Individuals with severe food and insect allergies should not rely totally on *Benadryl* but also must carry with them an injectable anti-anaphylaxis medication such as *Epi-Pen*.**

2. **Non-sedating antihistamines** Non-sedating antihistamines are now available both over the counter and by prescription. Examples of these include loratadine (*Claritin, Alavert*), desloratadine (*Clarinex*), cetirizine (*Zyrtec*), and fexofenadine (*Allegra*). They have the advantage of lasting twelve to twenty-four hours and have fewer side effects. They are definitely less sedat-

ing than *Benadryl. Zyrtec* may cause sedation in some people. Many are available as syrups or fast-dissolving tablets which young children will have no trouble taking. Ask your physician or pharmacist for help in deciding which medication is right for you and your child.

3. Pseudoephedrine nasal decongestant medication
This comes in many forms. Examples are:

- *Sudafed Children's Nasal Decongestant Liquid*
- *Sudafed Chewable Tablets*

These provide temporary relief from a stuffy nose due to a cold or allergy. These medications promote nasal and sinus drainage and may temporarily relieve sinus congestion and pressure but they often have unpleasant side-effects!

There are a variety of cough and cold medications on the market, which may help the nasal congestion due to colds and allergies. Most of these medications, like *Sudafed* mentioned above, have the potential for unpleasant side effects and have only limited benefit in alleviating the symptoms of a common cold. In contrast, allergy medications are far more effective in alleviating allergies. For further details on the management of colds and congestion, see the section on colds.

SUDAFED DOSING TABLE

Age	*Sudafed* Liquid 15 mg./5 ml.	*Sudafed Chewable Tablets* (15 mg./tablet)
6–12 months	Consult your physician.	
1–2 years	Consult your physician (an appropriate dose for a child heavier than 32 lbs. is ½ tsp. of liquid or ½ tablet every 6 hours).	
2–6 years	1 tsp.	1 tablet
6–12 years	2 tsp.	2 tablets
12 years and older	3–4 tsp.	3–4 tablets

Can be administered every 6–8 hours.

Note of Caution:

- Pseudoephedrine tends to make children and adults feel anxious and restless and may result in difficulty falling asleep.

- Pseudoephedrine may also cause palpitations, cardiac arrhythmias (irregularities of the heart beat), high blood pressure, and glaucoma.

- Use of *Sudafed* below two years of age is usually at the discretion of your physician. However, recommended doses for younger children are given above. Be careful: you may end up with a restless, nervous, and irritable child who will not or cannot settle down!

- Despite all the warnings discussed above, *Sudafed* may be useful in preventing earache during air travel, especially in a child or adult who is traveling with nasal congestion, a cold, or allergies. The medication should be given just prior to air travel and, during prolonged journeys, may be repeated every six hours as necessary.

4. **Topical nasal sprays** A variety of topical nasal sprays are available for treating colds, stuffy noses, and allergies.

   - **Nasal saline (salt water)**—this is ideal for clearing infants' noses, and for moisturizing dry noses, for example when flying. Nasal saline can be purchased commercially (*Nasal, Ocean Drops, Little Noses, Alta-mist*), or you can make up your own saline solution (dissolve ½ level tsp. of salt in 8 oz. of clean water).

- **Nasal decongestant drops or sprays.** Examples of these are *Afrin* or *Pseudoephedrine* nose drops (¼% or ½%). **These should NEVER be used for longer than five days!**

- **Steroid nose sprays.** These are very effective for treating nasal allergies and are available by prescription only. These are mentioned here for completeness sake and to remind you to take them along on your travels if your child suffers from nasal allergies.

5. **Epinephrine** This is an **essential** medication to have at home and on your travels if anyone in your family is severely allergic to bees or has severe food allergies. This medication is often supplied in a kit, the best known being *Epipen.*

Medications used to treat motion sickness

Examples of these are:

1. **Dimenhydrinate**—this comes as a liquid, chewable tablet, and tablet. A well-known preparation is *Dra-mamine* chewable tablets. These are fairly effective in the prevention and treatment of motion sickness. To prevent motion sickness, the first dose **should be taken one-half to one hour <u>before</u>** starting the activity that may induce motion sickness. Dosing is as follows:

DIMEMHYDRINATE (*DRAMAMINE*) DOSING TABLE

Age	Tablets (50 mg/tab)
2–6 years	1/4–1/2 tablet
6–12 years	1/2–1 tablet
12 years or older	1–2 tablets

Repeat every six to eight hours, as necessary.

Note of Caution:
- Should not be used below two years of age unless directed by a doctor.
- May cause drowsiness and interact with other sedatives, antihistamines, and alcohol.
- See the chapter on prevention and treatment of motion sickness in this book.

---

2. **Scopolamine patches** (*Transderm Scop*)—Are very effective in preventing motion sickness but their use is not approved below twelve years of age. A prescription is required for these patches.

3. **Homeopathic preparations**—See section on motion sickness in this book.

Medications to treat diarrhea

1. Oral Rehydration Salts

- Many commercially available powders can be mixed with drinkable water to make ideal solutions to prevent and treat dehydration associated with vomiting and diarrhea. Examples of these are *Kaolectrolyte,*

Ceralyte (which can be purchased by calling 1-888-237-2598), *IAMAT* oral rehydration solutions, and *Jianas Brother's Rehydration Powder*. Other preparations can be purchased as ready-made solutions, for example *Pedialyte* and *Liquilyte*. However, the ready-made liquid preparations are bulky and heavy. They are ideal for home use but may weigh too much to take with you on your travels.

- These solutions can be used safely at any age.
- See the chapter on vomiting and diarrhea in the book for the guidelines on the administration of electrolyte solutions.

Note of Caution:
- It is essential to make up the solution accurately, adding the correct amount of liquid to the powder (for example, one packet of Kaolectrolyte powder is added to 8 oz. of water).
- It is essential to use safe drinkable water (see preparation of drinkable water in this book).

---

2. *Imodium AD* *Imodium* chewable tablets may be used for treating diarrhea in older children and adults. Most episodes of diarrhea and diarrheal disease in children are **not** treated with any medication. Pay attention to maintaining hydration and preventing dehydration by the regular and appropriate use of electrolyte solutions as mentioned in the chapter on the treatment of diarrheal disease in the book. *Imodium,* in combination with certain antibiotics, may be very effective in treating travelers' diarrhea in older children and adults.

IMODIUM ADVANCED CHEWABLE TABLETS DOSING CHART

Age	DOSING (tablets) 1st dose	Next dose	Maximum number of tablets/day
6–8 years	1 tablet	½ tablet	2 tablets
9–11 years	1 tablet	½ tablet	3 tablets
12 years or older	2 tablets	1 tablet	4 tablets

Directions:
- Take the first dose after the first loose bowel movement.
- Take subsequent doses (half of the first dose) after each subsequent loose stool.
- Do not exceed the maximum recommended number of tablets per day.

Note of Caution:
- Imodium should **not** be used if your child has a high fever or blood or mucus in the stool.
- If the diarrhea persists, consult a physician.
- Not recommended for children below six years of age.
- May cause bowel obstruction in young children.
- As mentioned above, the mainstay in treating diarrhea in younger children is fluid therapy and **not** medication.

3. **Bismuth Subsalicylate (*Pepto Bismol*)** *Pepto Bismol* may also be used for the **prevention of travelers' diarrhea** as well as the **treatment of travelers' diarrhea.** (See section on travelers' diarrhea).

BISMUTH SUBSALICYLATE DOSING CHART

Age	*Pepto Bismol* Liquid	*Pepto Bismol* Chewable Tabs
Below 3 years	2.5–5 ml.	not recommended
3–6 years	5 ml.	⅓ tablet
6–9 years	10 ml.	⅔ tablet
9–12 years	15 ml.	1 tablet
>12 years	15–30 ml.	2 tablets

May repeat every 30–60 minutes to a maximum of eight doses in 24 hours.

NOTE: *Pepto Bismol* may color the tongue and stools black.

Medications for indigestion and heartburn

Examples of these are *Mylanta, Maalox,* and *Pepto Bismol.*

1. Mylanta chewable tablets

MYLANTA CHEWABLE TABLETS DOSING TABLE

Weight	Age	Tablets
Under 24 lbs.	Under 2 years	Not indicated
24 to 47 lbs.	2–5 years	1 tablet
48 to 95 lbs.	6–11 years	2 tablets
Greater than 95 lbs.	12 years and older	3 tablets

Directions:

- Maximum of three doses per twenty-four hours.
- Maximum of three tablets under six years of age or six tablets from six to eleven years of age during a twenty-four hour period.

Note of Caution:

- Consult a physician if indigestion persists.
- Do not use for longer than two weeks without consulting a physician.
- See section on abdominal pain in this book.

2. *Pepto Bismol* (see *Pepto Bismol* table above).

Laxatives and stool softeners

A variety of agents may be used to prevent and treat constipation. These include such simple measures as increasing water and juice intake, or using over-the-counter or prescription medications. Convenient medications to take along on your travels are:

1. Milk of Magnesia (MOM)

MOM DOSING CHART

Age	Dosage
Under 2 years	Consult a physician
2–5 years	1–3 tsp. once/day
6–11 years	1–2 tbsp. once/day
12 years and older	2–4 tbsp. once/day

Follow each dosage with a full glass (8 oz.) of fluid.

2. *Senokot* **liquid** A bowel action generally follows six to twelve hours after taking *Senokot*.

SENOKOT **LIQUID DOSING CHART**

Age	Dosage
Less than 2 years	Not indicated
2–6 years	½–¾ tsp
6–12 years	1–1½ tsp

Note:
• May give once or twice a day.
• If constipation persists, consult a physician.
• See the section on constipation in this book.

3. **Glycerine suppositories** Especially useful in infants. Keep suppositories in a cool location. One suppository is inserted into the rectum and the buttocks held together for one to two minutes. A bowel movement will usually follow shortly thereafter.

For easier administration, coat the glycerine suppository with *Vaseline* or *KY Jelly*. If the suppository has softened or melted due to warm temperatures, put it in the refrigerator prior to use to solidify it.

4. **Bisacodyl (*Dulcolax* suppositories)** The suppository is inserted into the rectum and the buttocks held together for one to two minutes. The suppository may be coated with *Vaseline* or *KY Jelly* to facilitate insertion. If the suppository has softened, place it in a refrigerator prior to use to solidify it. Usually effective within sixty minutes.

DULCOLAX SUPPOSITORY DOSAGE CHART
(5 mg./suppository)

Age	Number of Suppositories (Once a day)
Less than 2 years	Not indicated. Preferably use a glycerine suppository.
2–11 years	1 suppository
12 years and older	2 suppositories

Note of Caution:
• May cause abdominal cramps and rectal irritation.
• If constipation persists, consult a physician.

---

5. **Prescription stool softeners and laxatives** A variety of very effective and gentle medications are available to prevent and treat constipation. Examples of these are *Miralax, Kristalose,* and *lactulose*. These are available only by prescription. Ask your physician about these medications if your child is prone to constipation.

NOTE: Constipation in Children

- You should not rely on medication alone to treat constipation. Management of constipation should consist of the administration of appropriate fluids, a suitable diet, correct toilet habits, and stool softeners and laxatives if necessary. If constipation persists despite these measures, medical care should be sought. (See appropriate chapter in book.)

- Constipation tends to be a recurring problem and vigilance is necessary to prevent its recurrence.

- Constipation is a common problem while traveling. Plan ahead. Take stool softeners or laxatives with you on your travels. Drink plenty of fluids. Take regular bathroom breaks!

Ointments and creams.

1. **1% hydrocortisone cream or ointment.** This is used for the treatment of itchy rashes such as eczema (atopic dermatitis), insect stings and bites, and contact dermatitis.

NOTES OF CAUTION:

- Hydrocortisone (or any steroid cream) may make certain skin conditions worse, especially fungal infections such as ringworm and bacterial skin infections such as impetigo. If the rash does not improve, consult a physician.

- Do not use on the eyelids.

- Do not use for prolonged periods in the diaper area.

2. **Clotrimazole cream or ointment (*Lotrimin*).** This is used in the treatment of fungal infections of the skin such as ringworm, athlete's foot, and diaper rashes caused by yeasts.

NOTE OF CAUTION:
- If the rash does not resolve, consult a physician.

---

3. **Topical antibiotic creams and ointments.** Examples of these are *Triple antibiotic* ointment, *Neosporin* ointment (both over the counter) and *Bactroban* ointment or cream, which is only available by prescription.

4. **Diaper rash ointments and creams.** Essential if you have a child in diapers! Examples are *Desitin* ointment, *A&D* ointment and *Triple Paste* (especially effective).

5. ***Calamine* lotion.** Useful for insect bites and other rashes.

6. ***Vaseline*.** Ideal for:
   - The treatment of dry cracked lips, raw noses, and facial eczema.
   - Lubrication of thermometers and suppositories.

7. **Aloe vera gel,** for the treatment of burns.

Eye care.

Items that may be useful are:

1. **Artificial tears/eye drops.**
2. **Contact lens solution** (if necessary).
3. **Prescription antibiotic eye drops or eye ointments.**
4. **Saline solution.** This may be made up by dissolving ½ tsp. table salt in 8 oz. of clean water. Commercial saline eye drops may also be purchased. This is an ideal solution

for irrigating irritated eyes and for removing foreign bodies from the eye.

5. **An extra pair of glasses or contact lenses.** If your child wears eye glasses or contact lenses, do not forget to take an extra pair along on your travels.

6. **Sunglasses.**

Sun protection.

1. **Sunscreen.** Essential for the prevention of sunburn. Ideally use sunscreen with a sun protection factor (SPF) of 15 or greater. **Apply at least thirty minutes before exposure to the sun. Reapply often.** See section on sun protection.

2. **Lip balm** with a sun protection factor of 8 or greater.

3. **Sunglasses.**

Protection against insects.

1. **Insect repellents.** Preparations containing DEET are by far the most effective. Do not use preparations that contain more than 30% DEET in children. Recommended preparations for children are:

   a) **Sawyer controlled release insect repellant—** 20% DEET. This is probably one of the best preparations to use on children.

   b) **Ultrathon—33% DEET.** This is probably the most effective preparation overall and is ideal for adolescents and adults.

Notes of Caution:

- It is not generally recommended to use preparations containing greater than 30% DEET in children.
- DEET-containing preparations are extremely safe if used as directed.
- Do not apply to the fingers or hands of young children.
- Do not apply on cuts, wounds, or irritated skin. Do not put in eyes or mouth.
- See section on protecting your child against insect and tick bites, page 312.

2. **Insecticidal spray.** Sprays containing permethrin are used on clothing and mosquito nets. (See section on prevention of insect bites).

Dressings, bandages, and wound care.

1. Alcohol swabs for cleansing wounds.
2. Antibacterial towelettes for cleaning fingers, hands, and wounds.
3. *Betadine* or povidone lotion for sterilizing wounds.
4. Topical antibiotic ointment such as *Triple antibiotic ointment, Neosporin,* or *Bactroban.* (Listed under Ointments and Creams).
5. Band Aids.
6. Liquid band aids.
7. Sterile gauze swabs, 2 × 2 inches, and 4 × 4 inches.

8. Telfa dressing to apply directly to burns and other wounds. This will not stick to the wound.

9. *Steri-Strips* for repairing lacerations.

10. Butterfly band-aids for repairing lacerations.

11. Compound benzoin and tincture USP can be applied directly to the wound prior to applying the *Steri-Strip*. Allow the Benzoin to dry and then apply the *Steri-Strip*. This allows the *Steri-Strip* to attach to the skin more securely.

12. Gauze bandage to secure dressings.

13. Roll of adhesive tape to secure dressings, repair mosquito nets, fasten diapers, etc.

14. Ace (elastic) bandage.

15. Cold pack.

Instruments and other medical equipment.

1. Flexible digital thermometer for either oral or rectal use.

2. Metal tweezers.

3. Scissors.

4. Tick remover.

5. Five ml. medication dropper.

6. Large and small safety pins.

7. Latex-free protective gloves.

8. Bulb aspirator for sucking out mucus from noses and for irrigating ears and wounds.

9. Ziploc/plastic bags.

Optional additions to your medical kit.

These may be needed on hiking and camping expeditions or if traveling to tropical and underdeveloped countries.

1. Wet wipes.
2. Hand sanitizer gel.
3. Toilet paper and facial tissues.
4. A knock-down insect spray such as *Doom*.
5. Moleskin to prevent and treat blisters.
6. Athletes foot powder.
7. Water disinfection equipment.
8. Prescription antibiotics to be obtained from your child's physician. These may include antibiotics for treating ear infections, travelers' diarrhea, skin infections, etc. Antibiotic eye drops or eye ointment and antibiotic ear drops for swimmer's ear may also be a good idea.
9. Anti-malarial medication if traveling to a malarial area.
10. Survival wrap/thermal blanket.
11. Dental emergency kit.
12. Sterile needle syringe kit—recommended if traveling to countries where medical care and medical supplies are limited and the risk of transmission of AIDS and hepatitis are high.
13. Mosquito net.
14. Large collapsible plastic water bottle for storing water and making up oral rehydration solution.
15. N-95 face masks (if traveling to areas with outbreaks of SARS or similar contagious illnesses).

Sources of supplies

1. Travel Medicine Incorporated ((800) TRAVMED)
   www.travmed.com
2. Chinook Medical Gear ((800) 766-1365)
   www.chinookmed.com
3. SCS Ltd. (800) 749-8425 www.scs-mall.com

2

Traveling with Children

Anyone who has children will acknowledge that they change one's life! Remember this when making your travel plans.

Traveling with children poses unique challenges and requires much more planning than traveling without them. The stresses of travel escalate when you have a child in tow but so does the fun and enjoyment. You will probably have more laughs, but also more tears. Through the eyes of your child you will see the world in a very different way.

Travel often brings families closer together. Think back to your childhood. Aren't some of your most vivid and happy memories those vacations spent with your parents and siblings? These memories become even more precious once your parents are no longer with you. At the end of the day, the rewards of traveling with children are worth all the extra hassles, the extra effort, and the added stresses.

WHEN PLANNING YOUR TRAVELS, CONSIDER SOME OF THE FOLLOWING POINTS:

➢ The ages of your children.

Zero to three months

Home is the best place to be with a newborn. Traveling exposes us all to more infections. If an infant gets an infection and a fever in the first three months of life, you will need to find medical attention immediately. For this reason, it is better to wait until your baby is a little older before venturing far from home.

Four to twelve months

This may be a relatively easy time to travel. You have become used to your baby and the days of colic should be behind you.

You are in charge, which is not always the case when your child is older! Your baby has limited mobility and if you have a comfortable baby carrier you may not need a stroller.

Your baby may be breast-fed (the healthiest, easiest, cheapest, and most convenient) or formula fed. If formula fed, a source of safe water is essential. If you are unsure of the safety of the water supply, it may be easier to boil water once a day and store it in clean, sealed feeding bottles. Just before feeding, add the powdered formula. It is not necessary to reheat the formula. Discard any unused formula.

Bottles and nipples must be kept clean and can be sterilized by soaking in boiling water or in water to which a sterilizing tablet has been added. Ready-to-use formula is convenient but bulky and heavy. This may be a good choice if you are planning a very short trip.

Once your baby is eating solids, take along a supply of cereal and other baby foods. The foods you are familiar with may not be available in other countries.

Babies and toddlers require a lot of paraphernalia! Baby carriers, car seats, strollers, portable cribs, diapers, etc. The list seems endless. Take what you need, but do not economize with safety. An infant car seat is essential.

One to four years

This is probably the most challenging time to travel with children. They are usually more demanding, easily frustrated, and may be prone to temper tantrums. They are active, striving for independence on the one hand and yet totally reliant on their parents on the other. Their attention spans are usually short and they need to be entertained. Have you ever sat next to someone else's two-year-old on a long bus or plane ride?

- Children of this age require a more diverse diet and it is more difficult to provide safe food and water for them when traveling in developing countries. Always carry a supply of snacks, small boxes of juice, and plenty of wet wipes.

- Everything they lay their hands on is usually put straight into their mouths and you will have trouble keeping their hands clean.

- Until your child is potty trained you will need a supply of diapers. Disposable diapers usually make life easier but may not be readily available in developing countries. Always have a change of clothing easily accessible. Although one assumes life becomes easier once your child is toilet trained, this is not always the case. Young children need to "go now" and often have fixed ideas about where they will "poop." At times one longs for the diaper days!

• The equipment list you made for your infant is often even longer for your toddler! Toys that can be linked together make an adult's life a lot easier as less time is spent trying to retrieve or hunt for that "essential" toy beneath the aircraft seat or behind the bus seat.

Five years and older

As your children grow older, involve them in the planning of your trip. Let them help you research the places you intend to visit. Collect maps, brochures, visit the library or the bookstore, and search the web for information.

If you are traveling to another country, prepare your children for differences in culture and living conditions.

Children of this age should carry their own backpacks. Let them have some responsibility for what they choose but close supervision will be required. You may end up carrying the backpack if it is too heavy! Don't forget to include teddy.

➤ Your vacation location— deciding where to go.

Vacations that seem exotic and romantic when reading tourist brochures may be the exact opposite if you travel with children. Especially when traveling with young children, it may be sensible to stick to your tried and true vacation destination where there will be few surprises. The more exotic the location and the more off the beaten path, the greater the preparation and the greater the potential for disaster.

➢ Your expectations.

What do you expect from your vacation?

- Do you want to spend most of the time together as a family or do you feel you need time apart from your children?
- Do you want to stay in one location or do you want more variety?
- Is the purpose of your vacation relaxation or are you seeking stimulation and activity? Are you seeking a combination of these?
- Do you enjoy camping or does a luxury hotel have a greater appeal? What does your budget allow?
- Are you more comfortable revisiting a favorite and familiar place or do you want to try something completely different?
- Do you want to stay in your own country or are you ready for foreign travel?

Decide what is right for you and your family. Know your own limits. With the right attitude and realistic expectations, your vacation will be a success!

PACKING FOR YOUR TRIP

Travel with as little luggage as possible, but it is important to take along a favorite toy, blanket, etc. that will comfort your children and make them feel more secure.

When packing it is important not only to choose carefully **what** is packed but also **where** things are packed.

On plane and bus journeys, have a supply of snacks, change of diapers and clothing, etc. easily available. Plan to have sunscreen, insect repellant, and medications easily accessible but still in a safe place away from your toddlers inquisitive hands.

If traveling to a tropical or very warm country, cotton clothes are by far the coolest. Remember, although you may be tempted to pack just a tee shirt and shorts for your young children, it is wise to take long pants and long-sleeved shirts as well to help protect against sunburn and insect bites. One-piece sleep suits and special infant sleeping bags will help prevent infants and young children from insect bites at night.

Take comfortable, worn-in shoes. Include an extra pair of shoes in case one pair gets wet. It is often unsafe to walk barefoot in developing countries, not only because of injuries from glass or other sharp objects, but also to prevent parasitic infestations.

Don't forget to take a hat to protect your child from the sun. If traveling to a cold location, you will need something to keep his head warm. A baby can lose a lot of heat from his head. In cold climates, it is a good idea to dress in layers and have spare gloves and extra tights to keep your child warm.

MAKING YOUR JOURNEY MORE ENJOYABLE

- All of us are happier if not confined to a car or airplane or bus seat for long periods. If you are traveling by car, stop frequently to give children a chance to exercise and use a restroom.

- Provide toys, crayons, music, playing cards, etc. to entertain your children en route.

- Older children can use guidebooks and tourist bureau pamphlets to alert the family of upcoming places of interest. They can also follow along on a map and use a marker to trace the journey.
- Games like *I Spy* help pass the time and keep children aware of their surroundings.
- Encourage children to walk while waiting in an airport. They need to burn up as much energy when they can.
- Use the rest room just before boarding the plane. You may have to wait an hour or more after boarding before being able to leave your seat and the toilets on planes are tiny.

It is better to arrive late but safely and smiling!

CHOOSING YOUR ACCOMMODATIONS

- Consider safety and the ages of your children when choosing a place to stay.
- Make sure children are welcome. It is certainly not relaxing to constantly have to ask your child to be quiet or to worry that a priceless piece of furniture might be damaged.
- Consider upgrading your hotel accommodation to provide greater comfort for tired parents and children.
- A beach or a swimming pool is worth a great deal, but remember that children need constant supervision around water.
- Children need time to feel at home in a hotel room. Allow time and space for this.
- Many vacation resorts have "kid clubs" that offer supervised activities. This allows the adults time together while giving children the opportunity to make new friends. This is especially important if you have an only child.

PLANNING YOUR ITINERARY

- When traveling with children, **less is often more.**
- Do not plan to do too much. Allow time for unstructured play. A visit to the park for time to throw a Frisbee may be the highlight of the day.

    When we visited Disney World with our four-year-old, we all enjoyed the days more when we spent the afternoons at the hotel pool. By evening we were well-rested and ready to return to enjoy the fireworks.

- Plan your days so that there is something of interest for each of your children.
- Try to maintain your child's routine as far as possible. Try to plan excursions around your child's normal naptime.
- Museums, cathedrals, etc. may not hold a child's attention for long, but he will often discover something that interests him.

    Looking for lions in various shapes and forms kept our child alert and interested for hours when we spent an afternoon in St. Mark's Square in Venice. In Rome, our son found the antics of the cats on the grounds of the Coliseum infinitely more fascinating and entertaining than the ruins themselves.

- At times it might be sensible to let one parent have fun with the kids, while the other parent pursues more intellectual or strenuous activities.
- **Be flexible.**
- Memories of having fun feeding flocks of pigeons, tossing coins into a fountain or racing up the Spanish steps are more valuable and important than being able to say one

went to every Disney attraction or saw every cathedral in Paris!

SAFETY

Three important areas you should not neglect are car safety, water safety, and sun safety.

For further details, see section on safety during travel, page 78.

Flying/air travel.

Flying, especially in today's aircraft with cramped seating, is seldom restful or relaxing, but good planning might make the experience more tolerable. It has been said that there are only two classes of air travel: with children and without!

Here are some general tips to make the flight slightly less nerve-wracking:

- If possible, try to select less crowded flights. This is becoming increasingly difficult, if not impossible in this age of increased airline competition and cost-cutting! Friday evening and Sunday afternoon and evening flights are often overbooked and crowded. It is especially stressful to travel over Thanksgiving, Christmas, and New Year because they are very busy times.

- Having a seat for your child to stretch out on makes for a happier and more relaxed child and consequently a happier parent! Most airlines do not require booking a seat for a child below the age of two years. Regardless of age, it is preferable to book a seat for your child if you can afford it. This way, you can also bring along an airline-approved infant seat, which can double up as a car seat at your destination. When purchasing an infant car seat, try to purchase one that has a label that reads as follows: *This restraint is certified for use in motor vehicles and aircraft.* Choose one that is 16 inches or less in width as many coach seats aboard aircraft are only 16 inches wide. The car seat must be placed in a window seat so that it will not block the escape route in the event of any emergency. Children weighing less than twenty pounds should be placed rear-facing. From twenty to forty pounds your child should be in a forward-facing car seat. Children over forty pounds do not need to use a car seat but can be safely buckled up using the aircraft seatbelt. It is not safe to share an adult's seat belt by squeezing your child in between you and the belt. Most airlines will provide you with an extension for your seat belt if you are sharing your seat with a young child. Contact the airline for their policy on child restraint systems. For further information, you can also contact the FAA at 1-800-322-7873.

- Remember that injuries often occur when the plane hits air turbulence without warning and throws passengers from their seats. This is particularly likely to happen to an infant or a child, so booking your infant or young child their own seat is not only a comfort issue, but also a safety issue. Many infants and young children will cry and fuss more if confined to an infant car seat during a flight, so for these children using an infant seat during the flight may just not be practical. However, it is probably worthwhile using an infant car seat aboard the plane, even if your infant occupies his seat only when napping.

- If you are traveling long distances with an infant, try to reserve the seats just behind the bulkhead. Many airlines will then supply you with an infant bassinet or cot. If your children are slightly older, this might not be a good location as in many airlines these seats have armrests that do not fold back. This makes it difficult for a child to stretch out and sleep across you. The flickering images of the movie screened on the bulkhead may also make sleep even more difficult for you and your child.

- If you have a toddler, reserving an aisle seat is often a good idea as this will allow you and your toddler to take frequent walks around the cabin to ease the boredom and frustration of being confined to a seat for prolonged periods.

- Do not set out on your journey already sleep-deprived and exhausted. Do not leave too much to be done on the day of departure. Get a few good nights' sleep prior to departure and allow adequate time to get to the airport, check-in, clear security, and board the plane. This will ensure one "starts off on the right foot."

- Limit carry-on bags to essentials, but do not forget your child's teddy bear or favorite blanket, a supply of snacks, and boxes of juice.

- Carry essential medications with you.

- Prior to departure, prepare an activity pack with books, games, puzzles, and special treats to help entertain your child during the journey.

- Carry a change of clothing and sufficient disposable diapers for infants. Pack these items so that they are easily accessible during the flight.

- Children often get very thirsty during long flights so offer them liquids frequently.

- For young children who have graduated from a bottle, take along a "sippy cup" (trainer cup/cup with spout) to limit spills and sticky fingers.

- When making airline reservations, it is a good idea to reserve a child's meal, as children often do not appreciate the food served to adults. Adults may also not appreciate airline food! A hot dog or chicken nuggets may go down a lot better than a spinach quiche!

- Be careful when drinking hot beverages. Sudden movements can result in nasty burns.

- Do not let your children run in the aisles. This is not only inconsiderate towards other passengers and the flight attendants, but is dangerous. With air turbulence (and even without) young children may fall and injure themselves.

- Make sure carry-on luggage is safely and securely stored in the overhead luggage bins. Luggage falling from overhead bins is a common cause of injuries.
- Keep essential items under your seat to avoid having to repeatedly get up and search through the overhead bins.

HOW YOUNG IS TOO YOUNG TO FLY?

Parents frequently telephone our office and ask, "Can my child fly?" My wife, who gives telephone advice in our office, is often tempted to reply, "He can't walk yet, I would be surprised if he can fly!"

It used to be said that infants less than two weeks of age should not fly because of immature lungs. It is probably quite safe for healthy, full-term infants of this age to fly in today's pressurized aircraft. However, it is suggested you check with your pediatrician first. As discussed in the next chapter, the first three months are not a good time to travel because of the risk of acquiring infection.

Ears and flying.

Earache is common in people of all ages when flying. It is especially common in children. It is most likely to happen when the aircraft is descending just prior to landing. This is due to pressure changes within the middle ear and to the young child who does not understand what is happening, it may be alarming, as well as painful. Strategies to minimize this discomfort include:

- Allow an infant to nurse or suck on a bottle or pacifier during ascent and descent.
- Older children can be told to do the following—**on ascent,** hold the nose, close the mouth and suck in; **on descent,** hold the nose, fill the mouth with air, close it, and try to force the air through the closed nostrils.
- Chewing gum may help older children and adults, as this helps contract the muscles around the eustachian tube (the tube draining the middle ear), allowing it to stay open and equalize the pressure within the middle ear.
- If you know that your child usually suffers from severe ear discomfort when flying, it may be lessened by giving an adequate dose of ibuprofen or acetaminophen half an hour prior to flying. If the flight is long and sufficient time has elapsed, the dose can be repeated one hour prior to descent.
- If you or your child has nasal congestion from a cold, using an oral decongestant such as *Sudafed* prior to and during travel may help the nose and ears stay open. **Topical** nasal decongestants in the form of nasal sprays or drops can be particularly useful. Examples of these are *Afrin* and *Neo-Synephrine*. Ideally, these should be used half an hour prior to take off and half an hour prior to descent. They can be used either on their own or together

with oral decongestants. ⅛% or ¼% *Neo-Synephrine* may be used in infants older than six months of age (one to two drops in each nostril every four hours as necessary).

CAUTION

Nasal decongestant sprays should never be used for longer than five days.

- If you or your child is prone to nasal allergies or hay fever, using a steroid nasal spray for a few days before and during the flight will also help to decrease the swelling in the nose, ears, and sinuses. The swelling can be further relieved by using oral antihistamines such as diphenhydramine (*Benadryl*) or non-sedating antihistamines such as *Claritin, Clarinex, Zyrtec,* or *Allegra*. Parents should not take sedating antihistamines during flights if they will be driving a car after landing.

- Although it is often said that children who have an ear infection should not fly, there is no good evidence for this. Fluid in the middle ear may partially protect the child from some of the pain and discomfort experienced on taking off and landing. Infants and children with aerating (tympanostomy) tubes can also fly. Pain will be minimized as the tubes will equalize the pressure on either side of the eardrum. However, there is no doubt that flying with an acute cold with nasal and sinus congestion will be uncomfortable and may lead to a middle ear infection. This is the ideal time to use topical and oral decongestants. It may be a good idea to postpone your trip if at all possible.

- Cabin atmosphere contains very little humidity and mucous membranes dry out easily. Some of the crying and misery experienced by infants and children may be related to this discomfort. They can be nursed or offered other fluids frequently throughout the flight.

- Crying often helps unblock the ears. Distressing as this crying may be to you and to your fellow passengers, it often brings relief and a period of quiet!

- **It is never a good idea to try out any medication for the first time during a flight.** Many medications, especially cough and cold medications and antihistamines, may have unpleasant and unexpected side effects and may make your journey less pleasant. This is an understatement! **Always try a test dose of any medication a few days before you depart.**

Sedation and flying.

Generally speaking, it is not a good idea to sedate infants and children before a plane flight or other journey. A child sedative such as *Chloral Hydrate* and antihistamines such as diphenhydramine (*Benadryl*) or promethazine (*Phenergan*) may have the opposite effect: instead of ending up with a mellow and sleepy child, you may have an irritable, wide-awake, active child who cannot be pacified.

> *We made this mistake ourselves. We gave our three-year-old chloral hydrate to sedate him for a flight. He slept peacefully for two hours while the plane was held on the runway during a thunderstorm. He awoke as we took off. Our usually calm and pleasant little boy was transformed! For the next three hours we were the embarrassed owners of an uncontrollable, feisty, and badly-behaved child. Nothing calmed him. It was an unforgettable flight!*

If you feel you must try sedatives, discuss the issue with your child's physician prior to travel. Have a trial run several days before departure to assess the effect on your child. This will also enable you to establish the appropriate dose for your child. However, it should be reiterated that sedation is usually **not** a good idea and is **not** recommended during travel.

Jet lag.

Jet lag occurs when traveling across time zones. The body's internal clock and biological rhythms become out of sync with the new time zone or "outside clock." Jet lag is worse when traveling from west to east. The more time zones crossed, the more severe the effects. It is generally accepted that for each time zone crossed it will take at least one day for your body to adjust or recover.

On a ten-day vacation to East Asia, much of the time may be spent adjusting to jet lag because of the ten to twelve time zones crossed!

Symptoms include: insomnia, fatigue, irritability, poor concentration, and bowel upsets (especially constipation).

Jet lag is compounded by:

- Lack of sleep.
- The physical, emotional, and mental stresses of flying.
- Erratic and often unhealthy meals.
- Excess alcohol and caffeine ingestion.
- Irregular toilet habits.

Unfortunately, there are no wonder medications or remedies that work for all children or adults, but the following strategies may help:

- Be well-rested prior to travel. Try not to leave all of your travel arrangements and travel preparations until the last minute. Get to bed early and get a few good nights' rest in the days preceding your travel.

- Two or three days prior to departure try to schedule your activities closer to the time zone at your destination. For example, if traveling from west to east go to bed earlier and rise earlier.

- As you board the aircraft set your watch to your new time zone. Start adjusting your eating and sleeping habits to the new time zone.

- Keep well-hydrated during the flight. Drink plenty of water and other non-alcoholic beverages. Avoid alcohol and caffeine-containing products.

- Allow time to adapt to the new time zone at the other end of the flight. Do not arrange too hectic a schedule for the first three to five days if possible. European travelers often seek somewhere peaceful to spend a few days to relax and adjust to the new time zone. Non-retired American travelers, who typically get very little vacation compared to Europeans, do not enjoy this luxury as they typically schedule a trip over a brief holiday vacation, a child's spring break, or a one-week work reprieve. It is understandable that most Americans feel they need a vacation after the vacation! They do not recuperate from jet lag in either direction until several weeks after returning home!

- Force yourself to adapt to the new time zone as quickly as possible. Stay awake during daylight hours and go to bed at night.

- **Exposure to bright sunlight at the correct time of day** may hasten your adaptation to the new time zone. When traveling west to east, expose yourself to morning light. When traveling east to west, expose yourself to afternoon light. For example, when catching the late night flight from New York to London and arriving in London at 8 AM the following day, force yourself and your children to stay awake during the morning. Expose yourself to bright, outside light during the early part of the day. In the afternoon, avoid bright light, decrease activities and curtail caffeine-containing beverages and alcohol. Keep daytime naps short.

- Occasionally, parents may have to resort to sleeping tablets to help them sleep for a few nights in the new time zone. One adult should remain unsedated so that he or she can attend to the kids if necessary. A very effective sleeping tablet for adults is zoldipem (*Ambien*).

- It is usually **not** a good idea to sedate children. However, you may have to do this if your child is having a great deal of trouble falling asleep in the new time zone. A good children's sedative is *chloral hydrate.* This is a prescription medication and you should discuss this with your child's physician prior to departure. Some children may get sufficient sedation from an antihistamine such as *Benadryl* to enable them to go to sleep. Remember, these medications should always be given a trial run at home first. This may avoid unpleasant surprises on your vacation!

- Numerous other remedies have been tried. These include melatonin and a variety of herbal treatments. Melatonin, a hormone, has been shown to be effective in many studies. There are no studies in children so this cannot be recommended for them at present.

"Economy class syndrome"/ traveler's thrombosis/DVT.

You may well ask what a discussion on deep vein thrombosis/DVT (blood clot in the leg) is doing in a book on travel problems in children! Normal children rarely develop blood clots in their legs. However, children travel with parents and grandparents and it is a real tragedy if they become seriously ill or die from this largely **preventable** condition.

> *My mother in law developed a DVT and pulmonary embolus (blood clot to the lungs) after a long flight from the United States of America to South Africa. She spent some days in intensive care recovering from this avoidable condition. A few minutes of counseling, a pair of compression stockings and some leg exercises would have saved her weeks of illness and agony.*

The term "economy class syndrome" was originally used to describe a condition of blood clots in the legs that occurred in passengers during or after flying long distances in the coach section of the airplane. This is a misnomer as this condition can also occur in passengers in first class as well as in people traveling long distances by car, bus, or train. It may also occur after sitting for prolonged periods at a theater.

Small DVTs are not unusual after a long flight. Fortunately they seldom lead to major medical complications!

The tendency to develop blood clots in the legs on long journeys is due to a number of factors but especially:

- Immobility, which leads to sludging and pooling of the blood in the veins.
- Kinking of the blood vessels, related to the cramped position of the legs.

- Increased tendency of the blood to clot at high altitudes. Cabin pressure at cruising altitude is equivalent to an altitude of 6,000 to 8,000 feet.

Many other factors, such as those listed below, may also play a contributing role.

Risk factors for developing travelers' thrombosis include:

1. A history of blood clots.
2. Age: 40 years and older.
3. Obesity
4. Pregnancy
5. Recent surgery, especially orthopedic surgery to the legs.
6. Dehydration
7. Sedation
8. Certain diseases, especially blood diseases, heart disease, diabetes and malignancies.
9. Some drugs. Important examples of these are the birth control pill and tamoxifen (used in the treatment and prevention of breast cancer).
10. Recent excessive exertion, such as marathon running.

Many who develop DVT's after a flight do not have any of the above risk factors.

Prevention of travelers' thrombosis.

Traveler's thrombosis is a preventable disease! Below are some important ways that you can decrease the likelihood of developing traveler's thrombosis.

1. Move your legs often.
   - Extend your legs as far as possible, flex your ankles, pulling up and spreading your toes and then push down and curl your toes.
   - If there is not enough room to extend your legs, start with your feet flat on the floor and push down and curl your toes while lifting your heels from the floor. Then with your heels back on the floor, lift and spread your toes. Repeat this toe-heel cycle five times or more every thirty minutes.
   - Exercise your thigh muscles by sitting with your feet flat on the floor and slide your feet forward a few inches, then slide back and repeat.
   - Change your leg position frequently.
   - Get up and walk around the cabin as often as possible.

   Many airlines show a short film at the beginning of the flight describing the type of exercises you can do to minimize your risk of developing a DVT. Pay attention to this film. It may save your life!

2. Do not cross your legs, even for short periods.
3. Keep well hydrated. Drink plenty of water or electrolyte solutions such as *Gatorade* and other non-alcoholic beverages.
4. Limit alcohol intake and caffeine-containing beverages, all of which tend to lead to dehydration.
5. Avoid sedatives. These lead to more immobility.
6. Wear graduated compression stockings during the flight. These are extremely effective in preventing thrombosis. They are available at many drug stores.
7. Wear loose-fitting clothing.
8. Blood thinners/anticoagulants. These medications are recommended for certain high risk people. If you have

had a prior leg thrombosis, discuss the use of these with your doctor before traveling. They are not without risk and should not be started just before travel. Aspirin is **not** particularly effective in preventing venous thrombosis of the legs.

9. If traveling by car, stop frequently to stretch your legs.

Recognition and management of travelers' thrombosis.

The most common symptom of traveler's thrombosis is **calf pain** which develops during or soon after a long airplane flight. The pain is often mistaken for a muscle cramp. Other common symptoms are swelling of an ankle and later the development of a **cough, shortness of breath,** or **chest pain**. The chest pain may be so severe that it is mistaken for a heart attack. Rarely, a large clot breaks off, travels to the lung and causes sudden death.

If you develop any of the above symptoms, seek medical care promptly and **inform your physician of your recent journey** so that he/she may make the correct diagnosis.

NOTE: swelling of the ankles and feet is not unusual after a long flight.

For further information: www.airhealth.org/prevention

Motion sickness.

Children are more prone to motion sickness than are adults. It is especially common between four and twelve years of age. It occurs less frequently in the first two years of life.

The typical symptoms of motion sickness are nausea, vomiting, sweating, and increased salivation. Your child may also look very pale. A common symptom in younger children is an unsteady gait.

General measures to prevent motion sickness include:

- Avoiding dairy products and heavy and fatty meals.
- Giving your child a light meal three to four hours before your journey.
- Distracting your child by telling stories or letting them listen to music with headphones.
- Using medications to prevent and treat motion sickness.

➢ Road travel.

Car sickness may be minimized using these guidelines:

- If your child is older than twelve years, allow her to sit in the front seat.
- Focus on the horizon.
- Booster seats allow younger children to see out of the window.
- Keep the car well ventilated.
- Do not smoke in the car.
- Avoid video games and reading.
- Avoid tight clothing.

- Wearing dark glasses may help.
- If possible, avoid rough, winding, and hilly roads.
- Drive carefully and minimize rapid cornering, stopping, and acceleration.
- Try traveling at night.

If traveling by bus, sit towards the middle of the bus. Open the window slightly if possible.

Despite all these measures your child may still vomit. Have a plastic bag or container easily accessible. Wet wipes and a change of clothing are also a good idea!

➢ Air travel.

Most children do not develop air sickness when traveling in large commercial aircraft. These fly above the altitude of maximum turbulence and usually are fairly stable.

Measures to minimize air sickness:

- If possible, avoid small commuter flights which fly at low altitudes and are more prone to turbulence.

- Book seats over the wings. This is the most stable part of the aircraft.

- If your child feels nauseated encourage her to keep her head still and hold it firmly against the back of her seat.

- Keep eyes closed.

As mentioned before, have a container handy, as well as wet wipes and a change of clothing.

➢ Sea travel.

Sea sickness is more common than car or air sickness,

especially if traveling in small boats and across rough stretches of water.

Sea sickness may be minimized in the following ways:

- If traveling in a large ship, choose a cabin in the middle of the ship close to the waterline.

- If traveling by ferry, stay on the upper deck where there is ample fresh air. Focus on the horizon. If this is not possible, choose one of the lower decks close to the water line and near the middle of the boat. If possible, lie down and close eyes.

MEDICATIONS TO PREVENT MOTION SICKNESS

Sometimes the suggested precautions are inadequate and medication is needed to prevent or treat motion sickness.

Three medications commonly used in children are: diphenhydramine (*Benadryl*), dimenhydrinate (*Dramamine*), and promethazine (*Phenergan*). For the appropriate doses of *Benadryl* and *Dramamine* see the tables in the section "A Children's Medical Kit." Always consult the directions on the labels or manufacturers' packaging. Promethazine (*Phenergan*) is a prescription medication. Discuss the use of this with your child's doctor.

- These medications should be taken at least **half an hour before departure. It is easier to *prevent* motion sickness than to *treat* it.** During long journeys you will need to repeat the dose.

- *Dramamine* is not approved for children below two years of age.

- If you need to use medications such as *Benadryl, Dramamine,* or *Phenergan,* try these medications **prior** to your trip, as they may have unpleasant and unexpected side effects.

- Scopolamine patches are very effective in older children and adults. They are not approved below twelve years of age. Each patch lasts up to three days.

- Ginger is a homeopathic remedy that is moderately effective and very safe.

- Remember simple measures are often all that is necessary. Plan ahead and be prepared!

ACCIDENT PREVENTION WHILE TRAVELING

The dangers of travel are often exaggerated. This is aided and abetted by the media—aircraft accidents always make headline news. In fact, travel may be just as safe as staying at home!

Accidents are the leading cause of death among travelers under the age of fifty-five years. **Motor vehicle accidents** top the list, followed by **drowning**. People tend to exaggerate and worry about such unlikely dangers as airplane accidents and terrorism and to minimize the far more common dangers of motor vehicle accidents and drowning, both of which are preventable.

General safety.

Ground rules need to be established before departing and should be reinforced frequently.

- Dress your children in bright clothes so that they are easily visible.
- Pin a whistle onto the jacket of young children so that they can signal if they become separated from you.
- Decide on a meeting place in each location you visit, should you become separated.
- Young children should carry on their persons, cards listing their names, parents' names, and relevant contact numbers. This information should not be visible but carried in a safe pocket.
- Children should also carry on their persons cards listing the names and addresses of their hotels or motels.

This is also a good idea for parents to do, especially when in a foreign country!

- Parents should carry with them a recent photograph of their child.

- During wilderness travel, children should be taught to hug the nearest tree if they become lost.

- Teach children not to go anywhere with strangers.

- Teach children to identify the police, security guards, etc. These are the people they can ask for help.

- Travel inconspicuously. Do not wear expensive jewelry and watches. Do not flash money around. Teach your children to do the same.

- Keep valuables and travel documents in your room safe or your hotel safe.

Hotel safety.

Americans may be surprised when they realize that safety standards in many countries are not equivalent to those in the United States. This may be true even in good hotels in many western countries. Hotels may not have smoke alarms and may have dangerously unprotected balconies and windows that do not lock. Often one is able to open windows completely, even on very high floors where a fall may mean certain death.

When we traveled to Paris with our five-year-old son, we were shown to our room and immediately marveled at the spectacular view, which was seen through our floor-to-ceiling windows. We were somewhat alarmed when we realized that the window had no lock and there was no outside balcony or railing. It would have been quite easy for either an adult or a child to have opened the window and toppled out!

- Locate fire exits. Be able to locate them in the dark. Check that they can be opened from the inside and that they are not blocked off.
- Check new living and play areas from a safety point of view. Pay particular attention to windows, balconies, electrical outlets, and electrical cords.
- Do not allow children to play on the balcony.
- Never sit on the balcony railing! There have been many tragic deaths of holiday-makers falling to their deaths from balconies.

SAFETY IN THE BATHROOM

- Beware of hot water temperatures. In many hotels, the hotel hot water temperature is close to boiling! Severe burns can result.

Motor vehicle accidents.

- Always use seat belts. If renting a car, reserve a vehicle with seat belts. In many countries seat belts are not standard equipment on cars. Extra time and effort may be needed to locate a car with seat belts.
- Children less than four years of age need a car seat. Reserve one when booking a rental car or take your own.
- Older children may need a booster seat.
- Rent the largest car you can afford.
- Familiarize yourself with your rental vehicle. Get used to the controls. Don't just head out on to a busy highway. Drive around the car park a few times first.

- Avoid driving if fatigued. If you have just had a long flight, rest for a night or day before getting behind the wheel of a strange vehicle.

- Drive slowly. Roads may contain potholes and often are poorly signed. Local children may be playing on the roads. Animals may stray onto the road. Take extra care if the country you are traveling in drives on the other side of the road than yours.

- Avoid traveling at night, especially in rural areas and especially if you are unsure of the way.

- Do not drink and drive.

- Do not sleep in your car or RV at the roadside at night.

- Be very careful when stopping at scenic spots. In many countries these are prime targets for hijackers and thieves.

- Avoid traveling in open vehicles and in the back of trucks.

- Avoid overcrowded vehicles.

- Carrying children on motor bikes is especially dangerous! Don't do this! In fact it is better to avoid scooters and mopeds completely despite their obvious attraction. Scooter accidents and injuries are common, even in quiet resort locations. Don't be the sucker who keeps the local orthopedic surgeon in business!

- If traveling by taxi or if you have hired a driver, do not be afraid to tell your driver to slow down and drive more cautiously. Although the driver may appear very nonchalant and confident, his appearance may be misleading. Motor vehicle accidents occur with far greater frequency in developing countries where poor roads, poor vehicle maintenance, and poor traffic law enforcement are common.

- Insist upon safe behavior on sidewalks and when crossing roads. Traffic may be approaching from an unfamiliar direction.

Remember, vehicle accidents are the number one cause of death while on vacation or traveling!

Exposure to the elements.

Children are far more susceptible to extremes of temperatures, and special care should be taken in unusually cold or hot climates.

Hot climates:
- Increase fluid intake to maintain hydration.
- Wear appropriate clothing, including a hat with a wide brim.
- Use sunscreen.
- See the section on heat-related illness.

Cold climates:
- Hypothermia (a drop in body temperature) may occur in summer as well as winter, especially if one is wearing damp or wet clothing. Children lose heat very easily and heat loss is aggravated by windy conditions and excessive perspiration in rain-proof and wind-proof clothing.
- Change children's clothing as soon as it is wet.
- Dress appropriately. Dress in layers.
- Young children, especially infants, may lose a large amount of heat from their heads. A warm hat is essential.
- See the section on cold-related illness and hypothermia.

Walking and hiking.

When walking and hiking it is wise to wear closed shoes, not only to avoid bites from snakes but also to protect one-self from insect stings, sand fleas, and parasitic diseases such as hook worm. If walking in snake or tick-infested areas, it is a good idea to wear boots and long pants (see relevant sections for prevention and treatment of tick bites and insect bites and stings).

Swimming.

Drowning is the second most common cause of death while traveling.
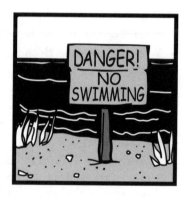
Swimming in unknown waters carries not only the risk of drowning but also the risk of acquiring water-borne diseases. These may enter directly through the skin or by swallowing water. Children tend to swallow much more water than adults while swimming and so are more prone to water-borne diseases.

Many swimming areas have dangerous currents and often there is no lifeguard on duty. Deserted beaches are often deserted for a reason! They may have dangerous cross currents, backwashes, and generally be unsafe for swimming. Find out from local people where it is safe to swim. Teach your children water safety.

Alcohol and swimming do not mix. You cannot supervise your children adequately if you have been drinking!

Holiday makers often try new water sports while on vacation. Get adequate instruction. If going snorkeling or scuba diving, always have a partner close by.

Many tropical waters contain a variety of poisonous fish and dangerous or even fatal stings may result. It is a good idea to wear rubber shoes or sandals when swimming in tropical waters. Ask the locals what the local hazards are.

In certain countries, sharks may be a problem. Rivers in Africa not only contain many parasitic diseases but also crocodiles and hippos! Hippos are responsible for many deaths in Africa.

Animal bites.

- Caution children about petting and playing with stray dogs and cats and other animals. They might not be as tolerant as the family pet back home and may carry rabies. Rabies is especially common in parts of Asia and Africa. (See section on animal bites and rabies.)
- It is a good general rule to tell your children never to approach or pet unknown animals even if they appear friendly. Watch, take photos, and don't touch.

Teenagers.

- Teenagers generally regard themselves as immortal and may be especially reckless when away from home.
- Many countries have a far more casual attitude towards alcohol than is present in the United States. **Adolescents and alcohol may be a lethal combination.**

- Adolescents love to partake in dangerous sports such as jet skiing, parasailing, scuba diving, etc. Alcohol should never be consumed around these sports. With the adolescent's typical belief in invincibility, he may venture out into unsafe waters. Constant vigilance is necessary!
- AIDS is a worldwide problem that shows no respect for class or age. In some areas up to seventy percent of prostitutes are HIV-positive. In Africa, a high percentage of the ordinary population is HIV-positive. **Body piercing** and **tattooing** carry the risk of acquiring Hepatitis B, C, and AIDS. Teach your teenagers to avoid all casual sexual encounters.

You will need to play the difficult role of, on the one hand being firm, but on the other hand also being understanding. Discuss your expectations and set clear-cut guidelines. Remember that just one sexual encounter or just one combination of a "holiday drink" and a swim may have a fatal outcome!

Other important safety tips.

- Avoid countries that are known to have drug-related violence or significant drug problems.
- Never purchase, transport, or use illegal drugs. Teach your children not to carry packages for strangers.
- Travel in groups, especially at night.
- Don't go out alone on beaches at night and never sleep on the beach.
- Camp only in designated campsites.
- If you intend to travel to locations where there is a possibility of political turmoil, it is an excellent idea to research the country of destination more thoroughly and learn of measures to safeguard you and your family.

Excellent sources for this are as follows:

1. *The Safe Travel Book* by Peter Savage.
2. *Travel Safely—at Home and Abroad* by Worring, Hibbard, and Schroeder.
3. Shorelands (800) 433-5256.
4. State Department Travel Warnings and Consular Information Sheets.

   Tel: (202) 647-5225 or (888) 407-4747. If outside the United States, call (317) 472-2328.
   Fax: (202) 747-3000

   Bureau of Consular Affairs Home Page:
   http://travel.state .gov.
5. The Department of State

   Tel: 202-647-4000 and ask to be connected to the desk covering your destination country.

Refer to other sections of this book that relate to accident prevention.

TRAVELING WITH CHILDREN OUTSIDE THE UNITED STATES

Travel, especially traveling abroad, is an enriching experience for both adults and children. Travel to foreign countries is one of the most important educational experiences a child can have and encourages all of us to become more tolerant of foreign customs and cultures.

Traveling with children is a lot more work and more stressful than traveling alone, but it can also be a lot more fun. Barriers erected by race and language often fall away in the company of children. Children are less inhibited than adults and often help break the ice. In many countries, when you travel with a child, the local population opens their hearts and homes to you and your family.

Traveling abroad can be as safe as staying at home if you are sensible about your choice of destination and if proper preparations and precautions are taken. Remote and primitive destinations are just not suitable for young children, particularly if you are traveling on a shoestring budget.

If you are planning to travel to remote and dangerous places **seek medical advice and information beforehand** about the hazards and dangers that you are likely to encounter there.

When one considers the risk of travel there are some **important differences between children and adults**.

- Whereas travelers' diarrhea is usually only an inconvenience to adults, young children may rapidly become dehydrated and require urgent medical attention.

- Children are more susceptible to extremes in environmental temperature. They more easily develop heat stroke and hypothermia.

- Children are more likely to get sunburned.

- Children are risk takers and often have poor judgment. They are more prone to accidents, drowning, animal bites, and poisoning.
- Some illnesses such as malaria, tuberculosis, and rabies tend to be more common and more severe in children.

Although most infectious illnesses that you acquire while traveling abroad cause symptoms while you are away, some (such as tuberculosis, malaria and some causes of diarrhea), may not give rise to symptoms until weeks or even months after you return.

Despite warnings about dreaded diseases, these are fortunately rare. Don't forget about motor vehicle accidents. They pose the greatest risk of death and serious medical problems during travel.

To prevent is better than to cure. For travelers, this is particularly important. **Most of the diseases and medical problems that people encounter abroad can be prevented.** The further afield you travel and the more remote and primitive your destination, the more important it is to be well prepared.

When traveling outside the United States, it is especially important to be honest with yourself about the level of discomfort and hardship you are willing to tolerate:

- Do you feel very insecure when you can't understand the local language?
- Do you feel that everyone should be able to speak English?
- Are you easily upset by uncertainty, unexpected delays and changes in your schedule?
- Does your anxiety level increase when you don't have access to medical care?
- Does unfamiliar food faze you?

- Do you need a hot shower every day?
- Does the absence of clean toilet facilities upset you?

Don't underestimate the psychological stress caused by lack of sleep, minor ailments (such as diarrhea, constipation, and skin rashes), strange food, lack of clean toilet facilities, and the inability to understand foreign languages.

It is vital to keep your sense of humor and not to overextend yourself.

Attitude is everything when you travel, especially when you travel with children. Minor mishaps may open doors to unexpected adventures and opportunities.

> *A family we met when we were hopelessly lost in Hong Kong showed us parts of the city the guidebooks would never have told us about!*

When traveling with children, less is often more.

Preparation for travel outside the United States.

- Preparation for travel is essential, especially with young children. Knowledge and preparation are the keys to a successful and medically uneventful trip. The extent of preparation depends not only on which country you visit, but also the location within the country. Are you traveling to large cities or to rural areas, to cool, dry areas or to humid tropical areas? The length and purpose of the journey will also influence your preparation.
- Learning more about the country you intend to visit, including its health problems, is wise. Involve older children and teenagers in this research. It can be fun as well as educational.

- Traveling to developing countries that lack clean water and disease-control programs requires specific preventative measures to avoid illnesses. Many of these measures are covered in this book. Additional sources for obtaining information on travel-related medical issues are listed below.

- Preparation is especially important if you plan to travel to countries with radically different cultures. You should prepare your children for different lifestyles and different standards of living. It may come as quite a shock to you and your children to witness the extent of poverty and disease in many developing countries.

- When traveling to remote, primitive or undeveloped areas it is especially important to have backup and evacuation plans. If you are traveling to remote locations, it would certainly be worthwhile for the adult and adolescent members of your party to take a first aid course before traveling.

Additional Sources of Information on Medical Issues Related to Foreign Travel

- *International Travel Health Guide* by Stuart R. Rose, is one of the best of the travel health guides and it is updated frequently It is recommended for the serious international traveler and contains a wealth of information on all aspects of travel. It can be purchased by calling (800) 872-8633. Internet at: www.travmed.com.

- Travellers' Health: *How to Stay Healthy Abroad* by Dr. Richard Dawood. 4th Edition 2002. An extremely comprehensive guide to travel and living abroad. Excellent!

- The Centers for Disease Control and Prevention (CDC). Fax information: (888) 232-3299. Voice information: (888) 232-3228. Internet at: http://www.cdc.gov. The CDC publishes an excellent book—*Health Information for International Travel,* which is available on the Internet or a hard copy can be purchased. This book is updated every two to three years.

- American Society of Tropical Medicine and Hygiene (ASTMH). Phone: (847) 480-9592. Internet at: http:// www.astmh.org. This society publishes a very useful booklet entitled, "Health Hints for the Tropics."

- International Society of Travel Medicine (ISTM), PO Box 871089, Stone Mountain, GA 30087. Phone: (770) 736-7060. Fax: (770) 736-6732. Internet at: http://www .istm.org.

- TRAVAX, 10625 West North Avenue, Milwaukee, WI 53226. Phone: (800) 433-5256. Internet at: http://www .tripprep.com. This is an excellent website with a wealth of information. It is highly recommended.

- Two pocket-sized books that are highly recommended if you plan to travel to exotic, lesser developed countries or undertake more serious adventure or wilderness travel are:

The Pocket Doctor, A Passport to Healthy Travel, by Dr. Stephen Bezruchka. This book contains a lot of common sense advice and sensitive sentiments regarding the environment and respect for other peoples.

A Comprehensive Guide to Wilderness and Travel Medicine, by Eric A. Weiss, M.D., has a wealth of practical advice for handling medical emergencies where medical care is not readily available.

The pre-travel medical consultation

A pre-travel consultation and examination by your physician or at a travel clinic is recommended for *everyone* who plans an extended stay in a developing or tropical country. Ideally, this visit should be eight to twelve weeks before departure to allow sufficient time for the special vaccinations recommended for some countries. However, even if you think you have left it too late, a visit just prior to your departure is still worthwhile.

NOTE: Your own physician or your child's pediatrician may not be familiar with the latest health recommendations for travel to countries outside the United States. **It is definitely worthwhile consulting a specialist in travel medicine or an infectious disease physician if you intend to travel to developing, tropical, or subtropical countries.**

LOCATING A TRAVEL CLINIC OR A TRAVEL MEDICINE PHYSICIAN.

Most teaching hospitals and many community hospitals have travel clinics. The following sources can also help you locate a travel medicine clinic in your area:

- International Society of Travel Medicine (ISTM)
  Website: http://www.istm.org
- American Society of Tropical Medicine and Hygiene (ASTMH)
  Website: http://www.astmh.org/clinics/clinindex.html
- Shoreland's Travel Health Online
  Website: http://www .tripprep.com
- Travel Medicine, Inc.
  Website: http://www.travmed.com

The cost of consulting a travel clinic and the immunizations that you and your child may require are not insignificant and may **not** be covered by your medical insurance. However, this will be money well spent because the consequences of diseases such as malaria and hepatitis are far greater. Consulting a travel medical specialist will also help you to avoid accidents, to make wise choices regarding safe food and water, and guide you about the many complex issues that you may encounter. The travel clinic will also advise you about medications you should take with you to prevent and treat travelers' diarrhea, malaria, motion sickness, acute mountain sickness, etc.

If you intend traveling to a country that has a signifi-cant risk of tuberculosis, all members of the family should have a **tuberculin skin test** prior to departure. This test should be repeated when you return.

HOW YOUNG IS TOO YOUNG TO TRAVEL?

- It is unwise to travel to developing countries with infants who are less than six months of age. The pri-mary immunization series is not complete and it is more difficult to prevent and treat insect-borne illness-es such as malaria in this age group.
- Many immunizations recommended for travel cannot be given to children below two years of age. The immu-nization against typhoid is one example.
- Diarrheal illness also tends to be more severe in infants and young children and is more likely to lead to dehy-dration.
- The younger the child, the harder it is to assess the degree of illness. Children below three years of age can-not localize pain or explain their symptoms well. Diag-nosis is often difficult and young children may become very ill very quickly.

Some authorities hold the more extreme view that is prefer-able not to travel to developing countries with children younger than age three because of the risk of travelers' diarrhea, tuberculosis, and malaria. This is sane advice if you intend to travel to a country that has a drug resistant type of malaria (chloroquine-resistant falciparum malaria).

IMMUNIZATIONS

Recommending appropriate vaccinations for travel is extremely complex. For this reason it is advisable that you consult a travel clinic or travel medicine physician or infectious disease physician to ensure you receive accurate information and the correct immunizations.

Many of these vaccinations are expensive and their cost may not be covered by your medical insurance. An experienced travel clinic physician can help you evaluate the cost benefit ratio and advise you as to which are the most important immunizations to receive.

Remember that immunizations against infectious diseases are one of the most important medical advances made and may save you and your child serious illness and even death. There are no cures for many of the illness which immunization prevents. Antibiotics are not effective against measles, hepatitis, rabies, and many other vaccine-preventable diseases.

NOTE: Travel is also a good time for adults to update their routine immunizations.

Immunizations fall into three categories: routine, recommended, and required.

➢ *ROUTINE* IMMUNIZATIONS

These are the immunizations most children routinely receive during infancy and childhood as part of their normal preventive health care. **Make sure your child is up-to-date with these routine immunizations,** because many of the diseases that these immunizations protect against are still prevalent in other parts of the world. These routine immunizations may be even more important than the travel immunizations discussed later in this section. **It is foolhardy to skip these routine immunizations if you plan extensive travels outside the United States with your child, especially to developing countries.**

The routine preventive immunization schedule varies from country to country and even in the United States is frequently updated and changed.

Immunization schedules can be modified and accelerated if traveling to foreign countries, especially if a trip is being planned to a developing country. For example, your child's first measles immunization may be given as early as six months of age and repeated at one year of age.

DTaP.

Diphtheria vaccine, Tetanus, and Pertussis (whooping cough) vaccines are usually combined into one vaccine known as the DTaP. The DTaP may also be combined with other vaccines in the same shot.

Once the primary DTaP vaccination series is complete, tetanus/diphtheria (Td) boosters should be given every ten years. In certain circumstances, for example after a contaminated wound, an additional dose of Td may be required to prevent tetanus. Because you cannot guarantee that your child will not get a contaminated wound while you are traveling, a Td booster is recommended every five years.

Diphtheria boosters are recommended for all travelers to the Russian Federation, Ukraine, and Tadjikistan, and for long-term visits (more than four weeks) to Africa, Asia, and South America.

Polio vaccine.

In the United States, this vaccine is given as an injectable vaccine known as the IPV. In many countries, the oral polio vaccine (OPV) is still used. A one-time booster of IPV is recommended for travelers to developing countries.

Measles/Mumps/Rubella (MMR) vaccine.

Measles is still common in many developing countries and is a common cause of childhood death in these countries.

Measles may cause a severe life-threatening illness, even in well-nourished, otherwise-healthy children.

Haemophilus Type B (HIB) vaccine.

This vaccine prevents illnesses due to the *Haemophilus* Type B bacterium. This bacterium was a common cause of pneumonia and meningitis in the United States. These illnesses are still common in many countries.

Hepatitis B (Hep B) vaccine.

For details see below.

Varicella (chicken pox) vaccine.

Pneumococcal vaccine.

The bacterium *streptococcus pneumoniae* is the most important bacterial cause of ear infections (otitis media) and sinusitis in most parts of the world, including the United States. It may also cause pneumonia, severe blood stream infections (septicemia), and bacterial meningitis.

New combinations of the above vaccinations become available almost every year. The bottom line is that your child needs to be protected against diphtheria, tetanus, whooping cough (pertussis), polio, measles, mumps, rubella, *Haemophilus* Type B disease, hepatitis B, chicken pox (varicella), and Pneumococcal disease!

➢ *RECOMMENDED* IMMUNIZATIONS

Some of these immunizations are often recommended even if you do not intend to travel

Hepatitis A vaccine.

- **Hepatitis A is the most common vaccine-preventable disease that affects travelers.** This is an extremely important vaccine, especially for adults.
- This vaccine can be given to children above two years of age. Children below two years of age can be given immune globulin to prevent hepatitis A.

Although travelers frequently worry about acquiring cholera or typhoid, they are far more likely to acquire hepatitis A. Hepatitis A can cause severe liver disease and even death in adults, especially in the older population. It's not unusual for children to acquire hepatitis A and not show any signs of significant illness; however, they may pass hepatitis A on to their parents or grandparents who may become seriously ill. **It is foolish to forgo receiving this very effective vaccination!**

Hepatitis B vaccine.

- This vaccination is recommended for everyone.
- Not all children and adults will have received the hepatitis B vaccine as part of their routine immunization series in childhood.
- Hepatitis B is a preventable disease that can lead to severe liver disease later in life, including cirrhosis of the liver and liver cancer.

Individuals, who have received neither the hepatitis B nor the hepatitis A vaccine, can be given a combination vaccine (*TWINRIX*).

Typhoid vaccine.

- Typhoid fever is a hazard in some developing countries.
- The typhoid vaccine may be given orally or as an injection. Children above six years of age and adults may

receive the oral vaccine. Children from two to six years of age should receive the injectable vaccine.

Influenza vaccine.

- This is recommended if you are traveling over the winter months, especially if your child has a chronic disease such as asthma or heart disease.
- Different countries have outbreaks of influenza at different times of the year. Check before departing. The southern hemisphere has its flu season between April and September. Outbreaks may occur year-round in the tropics.
- If your child has not had a flu shot before, he or she may need two shots at least a month apart.
- The influenza vaccine is recommended for many children and adults, even if not traveling.

Other vaccines.

Other vaccines that fall into the group of recommended vaccines include those against Japanese encephalitis, rabies, meningococcal disease, plague, and tick-born encephalitis. In many parts of the world, especially southeast Asia, rabies poses a significant risk, particularly to children. Rabies vaccine is recommended for children who will be spending many months in an area where rabies is prevalent.

➤ *REQUIRED* IMMUNIZATIONS

A required vaccination is one that is required for entry into certain countries.

Yellow fever vaccine.

- At present, the only vaccination officially required for entry into some countries is that for yellow fever.

- Yellow fever may be a severe and a sometimes fatal illness that is caused by a virus transmitted by infected mosquitoes.

- This vaccine can only be given by special travel clinics. It is not recommended for children under six months of age.

- **Many countries require a valid yellow-fever vaccination certificate for entry of travelers older than one year of age.** Ask your travel physician or travel agent if you need this vaccine. Proof of yellow fever vaccination should be recorded on the International Certificate of Vaccination (also know as the **"Yellow Card"**).

Cholera vaccine.

The cholera vaccine is not very effective and is no longer recommended by the World Health Organization (WHO) for travel to cholera-endemic areas. However, you may be unlucky enough to come across a border official who insists that cholera vaccination is required for entry into the country. Therefore it is recommended that you obtain a medical waiver. This should be written on official-looking paper and have an official stamp and signature.

If you do not have an appropriate certificate documenting that you or your children have had the yellow fever or cholera vaccine or do not have a medical waiver, you may have to be vaccinated at a border post where the sterility of the syringes and needles cannot be guaranteed.

DENTAL CHECKUP

A visit to your dentist is a good idea if you are planning a long stay in a developing country. Arrange this visit well in advance to allow sufficient time to get all necessary dental work done. Good dental care may be hard to find in lesser developed countries. Sterility might not be maintained for dental procedures, thus increasing the risk of severe infections such as HIV-infection, hepatitis B, and hepatitis C.

- Many children with congenital heart defects require antibiotic prophylaxis when they receive dental treatment. These children should take along a supply of an appropriate antibiotic.
- If you are likely to need dental care or are planning a long stay in a developing country, you should take with you a supply of sterile syringes and needles or even consider purchasing a dental kit from an appropriate commercial source (for example, Travel Medicine Inc.: (800) TRAV-MED or Chinook Medical Gear: (800) 766-1365). Discuss this with your dentist.

EYEGLASSES

- If you or your child wears contact lenses or eyeglasses, take a spare pair with you.
- Keep a copy of eyeglass prescriptions with you.
- It is a good idea for anyone who wears contact lenses to also take along a pair of eyeglasses in case they develop an eye infection, e.g., conjunctivitis (pink eye). If this happens it is important not to wear contact lenses until the infection has cleared.
- It is also a good idea to ask your physician or eye doctor for a prescription for antibacterial eye drops to take with you.

DOCUMENTS, PASSPORTS, VISAS, ETC.

- Photocopies should be made of all important travel documents. You should carry a copy, file one at home, and leave one or two sets with people you can trust as emergency contacts. Copies should not be left in luggage to be lost or stolen!

- Carry tickets, passport, and traveler's checks on your person while traveling. At your destination, it may be wiser to leave passports and plane tickets in the hotel safe.
- Travelers should assume that pickpockets are everywhere.

Passports

- Each family member must have his or her own passport. **Check the expiration date to make sure all the passports are valid for the duration of the trip.**

  My wife researched these services recently. She discovered just two days before we were leaving for South Africa that our son's passport had expired! This discovery was a life-shortening experience for her! Our family relies on her organizational skills for tickets, passports, and visas. A desperate phone call to our travel agent produced the name of a company that would expedite passport renewals. The next few hours were spent writing large checks and soon the passport, a handful of forms and new photographs were on their way to the west coast. The precious passport was returned just thirty minutes before we left for the airport. No Fedex van has ever received a greater welcome at our home! What a tribute to American efficiency!

- Allow six to eight weeks when applying for a new passport or renewing an old one. Specialized passport services are able to obtain passports at much shorter notice but at far greater cost. An example of such a service is American Passport Express, tel: (800) 841-6778, Internet at http://www.americanpassport.com.

Visas

You and your children will need visas to visit some countries. A visa is obtained from the embassy or consulate of the country you intend to visit. It allows you to enter the country and stay for a specified time.

- If you are visiting a number of countries, it may take some time to get all the required visas, so allow adequate time for this processing.

- Check with your travel agent or contact the embassy of the countries you intend to visit, or write to Passport Services, US Department of State, Washington, DC, 20524. Another source for obtaining information about visa requirements is the web site of the Bureau of Consular Affairs at http://travel.state.gov/foreignentryreqs.html.

Double check any information you are given about visas.

My wife travels on a South African passport and was told she did not need a visa to visit Italy. En route to Rome we had a stopover in Brussels. It was here the "fun" began. The customs official said, "You have a small problem. You do not have a visa for Belgium." She explained that we were en route to Rome and did not intend to leave the Brussels airport. The official's face tightened and he announced that we now had a "big" problem! "Where is the visa for Italy?" he asked. We were escorted to a holding room to await an interview with a senior immigration official. He courteously stated that my wife should not have been allowed to board the plane in the United States without a visa for Italy. He said she would have to return to the United States on the next flight out of Brussels. Our son and I would be permitted to continue to Italy!

Our seven-year-old was devastated by the thought that Mummy might have to go home. Big tears trickled down from under his Harry Potter glasses and he said, "But Mum, it is your birthday." We saw the immigration officer's eyes glance down at my wife's passport and his expression softened for just a second. "Return to the waiting room and I will see what I can do."

The next hour was spent in the company of two men traveling with forged passports and a suspected drug dealer who was in handcuffs. This was enough to impress upon us the seriousness of my wife's predicament.

Finally we were summoned back into the interview room and my wife was handed her passport which now sported two new visas, one for Belgium and one for Italy. Also in the passport was a note which read, "Happy Birthday, from the Belgian immigration authorities."

Custody Papers

Single parents should carry copies of custody papers in case questions arise when crossing international borders with a child, especially when the child has a different last name. Some countries require a certified letter from the other parent giving their consent for the child to cross borders.

PERSONAL MEDICAL INFORMATION AND MEDICATIONS

- If anyone in your family has a complex medical illness, photocopies of the relevant medical records should be carried with you. This record should include a complete list of medications with their correct pharmacological names, because the trade names of the medications vary from country to country. Take copies of all prescriptions with you. It is also a good idea to take along a letter from your child's doctor listing medications she is on and their dosage. Such a letter is essential if you are carrying syringes and needles.

- Medicines should be carried in their original containers.
- **Keep medications with you in your carry-on luggage.** Medicines should **not** be left with your checked luggage, which may be separated from you for prolonged periods or be lost.
- Emergency medications such as Epinephrine kits (*Epipen*), asthma medications, seizure medications and diabetic medications (insulin, glucagon, and syringes) should **always** be easily accessible.
- It is a good idea to take along **extra** medications in case of unscheduled delays.
- Do not forget to take along your medical kit.

HEALTH INSURANCE

It is often stated that if you can't afford travel insurance you can't afford to travel! This would deprive many people of the excitement and advantages of travel and may be a somewhat extreme point of view. Be sensible, and especially if there is anyone in your party with a significant medical condition (or any elderly people), make sure you purchase supplemental travel insurance.

The first step is to determine if the medical insurance that you have for care in the United States will cover medical expenses incurred while outside the country. Check the small print in your health insurance policy, and phone your medical insurance company and confirm what services will be covered. Have this put in writing.

Travel insurance

There are many types of travel insurance and your travel agent may be able to guide you in finding appropriate coverage. The best type of **travel insurance is travel insurance with assistance.** The amount of coverage you need will depend on where you are going, how long you will be there, and the health of the members of your party.

Two sources of travel insurance with assistance are:

Travel Assistance International
9200 Keystone Crossing
Suite 300
Indianapolis, IN 46240
(800) 821-2828

TravMed-Medex
Box 10623
Baltimore, MD 21285
(800) 732-5309

There are many other excellent companies that provide similar services.

Evacuation insurance is separate from health insurance and should be considered for travelers with specialized medical problems or when visiting especially remote and dangerous parts of the world. Injuries sustained during motor vehicle accidents are the most likely reason travelers may require evacuation.

Your travel agent should be able to guide you in obtaining evacuation insurance. Different companies provide services in different parts of the world, and you will need to research this before you depart. Dr. Stuart Rose's book, *International Travel Health Guide* is an excellent source for a number of companies which specialize in air ambulance services.

FINDING HEALTH CARE WHILE TRAVELING

Before traveling, especially if traveling to lesser-developed countries and out of the way places, stop and think what you would do if one of your family or party became ill or disabled while traveling. If you have a well thought-out plan and appropriate phone numbers and addresses, you are less likely to panic and will be better able to cope with the situation.

Many people born and brought up in the United States are inclined to think that the United States is the only country in the world capable of providing good medical care. This is simply not true. The standard of medical care in many countries may be just as high as that in the United States. This applies particularly to England, western Europe, Canada, Australia, New Zealand, many Asian countries, and South Africa.

The medical facilities in some countries may appear less modern and sophisticated than in the United States and often don't meet the same hygiene and cleanliness standards. However, the physician taking care of you may have far greater expertise in tropical diseases such as malaria and typhoid than your physician back home. It is natural to feel insecure in a strange environment and the following are some suggestions for obtaining medical care when traveling:

Local Contacts. Ask yourself if you know anyone locally (for example, a member of the expatriate community) who can recommend a good physician.

Hotels. If you are staying in a hotel, the hotel staff may be able to recommend a doctor who may even visit you in your room. Alternatively, they may be able to refer you to a reputable clinic or hospital in the vicinity.

Embassy or consulate. The United States embassy or consulate will often be able to recommend local physicians, clinics, hospitals, etc.

International Association of Medical Assistance to Travelers (IAMAT). IAMAT is established throughout the world. Members can call and be referred to a local physician who speaks the traveler's native language. To access the service, the traveler must be a member of IAMAT. The address is 417 Center Street, Lewiston, NY 14092 and the phone number is (716) 754-4883. Contact IAMAT before you travel and consider joining this organization. There is no charge to join IAMAT but a donation will be gratefully acknowledged. This organization will provide you with a booklet of recommended physicians in different countries as well as other useful information for your travels.

Personal Physicians Worldwide. This organization provides truly excellent service but is very expensive. If you plan extensive travels, and a member of your family has a medical problem, and you can afford these services, this is the organization to contact. The address is 815 Connecticut Avenue NW, Washington DC 20006. Their Website is http://www.personalphysicians.com.

Remember, **to prevent is better than to cure.** For travelers, this is particularly important. **Most of the diseases and medical problems that people encounter abroad can be prevented.** The further afield you travel and the more remote and primitive the location, the more important it is to be well prepared.

As mentioned earlier, if traveling to remote locations, it will certainly be worthwhile for the adult and adolescent members of your party to take a first aid course before traveling.

POST-TRAVEL PHYSICAL

A post-travel physical with your child's doctor is a good idea if:

- Your child has been ill while away.

- Your child has diarrhea lasting longer than ten days or diarrhea that recurs.

- Your child develops an **unexplained fever.** Remind your child's doctor that you have traveled recently and give him details of where you have been. This is especially important if you have traveled to areas where malaria is prevalent. Insist on a blood test to exclude malaria and have these tests repeated if your child remains ill. Most people who acquire malaria on their travels do not develop symptoms until they have returned home.

- You have traveled to an area with a high incidence of tuberculosis you should have a tuberculin skin test six weeks after returning home.

- You or your child develops unusual symptoms after traveling, especially if you have been to tropical or developing countries. **Do not delay** this visit to your doctor. If your symptoms persist, **insist** on a referral to an infectious disease specialist or a physician who specializes in travel-related illnesses.

SUMMARY

Despite the hazards discussed above, traveling abroad can be safe if one is sensible and takes appropriate precautions and preventive measures. Do not let these hazards deter foreign travel as the positive aspects of travel usually outweigh the negative ones.

Remember that most travelers return home quite safely without having had any serious illnesses. Remember, also, that most travel illnesses and accidents can be prevented.

TRAVELERS' DIARRHEA

Refer also to:
Preparation of safe food and water, page 129.
Diarrhea and dehydration, page 257.

AN OVERVIEW

What is it?

Who gets it?

What causes it?

How do you get it?

A. *Prevention* of travelers' diarrhea

1. General preventive measures
   - Hygiene
   - Liquids
   - Foods
2. Medications to prevent travelers' diarrhea

B. *Treatment* of travelers' diarrhea

1. Infants and children less than three years old
   - Mild diarrhea
   - Moderate to severe diarrhea
2. Children older than three years of age and adults
   - Mild to moderate diarrhea
   - Moderate to severe diarrhea

Points to note with fluid and nutritional therapy.

Using medications to treat travelers' diarrhea.

Differences between "usual" diarrhea back home and travelers' diarrhea.

When to seek medical care.

Homemade electrolyte solutions.

SUMMARY OF THE PREVENTION AND TREATMENT OF TRAVELERS' DIARRHEA

1. If you are traveling to a lesser-developed country, there is a good chance that someone in your party **will** get travelers' diarrhea—**be prepared for it!**

2. **Visit** your physician or travel clinic before you depart to discuss the prevention and treatment of travelers' diarrhea. If recommended, get prescriptions for antibiotics for travelers' diarrhea. Purchase the antibiotics, *Pepto Bismol,* and *Imodium* and know the dosages for each member of your party.

3. Pay attention to the general preventive measures for travelers' diarrhea, regarding hygiene and liquid and food precautions.

4. Consider taking *Pepto Bismol* prophylactically (preventively).

5. Drink extra fluids at the first sign of diarrhea.

6. If diarrhea develops, consider taking antibiotics and/or *Imodium*.

7. Watch out for the symptoms and signs of dehydration.

8. Continue drinking extra fluids until the diarrhea has stopped.

9. Know when to seek medical care.

Travelers' diarrhea—what is it?

Travelers' diarrhea is by far the most common travel-related illness you are likely to acquire while traveling in lesser-developed countries.

Travelers' diarrhea is diarrhea that occurs in the context of travel. Travelers' diarrhea is especially common in the first week of travel, but it may develop at any time during a trip or even after returning home. A person with travelers' diarrhea has frequent, loose bowel movements, abdominal cramps, nausea, and sometimes vomiting. Fever may also be present. Repeated bouts of travelers' diarrhea may occur, so having one bout of travelers' diarrhea does not immunize you or prevent you from getting it again.

In adults, travelers' diarrhea usually lasts three to four days, but this may be enough to ruin a carefully planned vacation or business trip. In children, travelers' diarrhea frequently lasts longer than a week. **Children younger than three years of age are especially prone to a more severe form of travelers' diarrhea which carries an increased risk of dehydration.** The elderly are also more prone to developing dehydration.

Who gets travelers' diarrhea?

Anyone can get travelers' diarrhea but it is more common in children than in adults. It is especially common in adolescents and in children below two years of age. **At least half of the people who travel from an industrialized country, such as the United States, to a developing country will experience travelers' diarrhea.** The chances that you or your child will develop travelers' diarrhea will depend on which countries you visit, how long you stay there, and the precautions you take to prevent it. Individual factors such as a lack of immunity and the presence of certain bowel diseases may predispose you to the development of travelers' diarrhea. If you are prone to bowel disturbances, be sure to maximize your preventative measures.

The world can be divided into three zones according to the risk of getting travelers' diarrhea:

- Low risk areas—the United States, Canada, Northern and Central Europe, Australia, New Zealand, and Japan.
- Intermediate risk areas—Mediterranean countries, the Caribbean, South Africa and Korea.
- High risk areas—the rest of the world.

What causes it?

A wide variety of bacteria, viruses, and parasites cause travelers' diarrhea. Most cases of travelers' diarrhea are due to bacteria. Very serious causes of diarrhea that may be acquired while traveling include cholera, typhoid, and amebiasis. Dysentery, diarrhea with blood and mucus in the stool, frequently accompanied by high fever and severe abdominal pain, may be caused by typhoid and amebiasis. Fortunately, these illnesses are rare. Cholera may cause life-threatening diarrhea. It is definitely advisable not to travel to areas of the world experiencing cholera epidemics.

How do you get travelers' diarrhea?

Travelers' diarrhea is acquired by eating contaminated food or by drinking contaminated water or other beverages, or by eating with dirty fingers or hands. Most travelers' diarrhea acquired while traveling abroad is due to eating contaminated food. However, if you get diarrhea while backpacking or camping in the wilderness in the United States, it is more likely that you acquired it from contaminated water.

A. *PREVENTION* OF TRAVELERS' DIARRHEA

It is extremely difficult to prevent travelers' diarrhea, but the chances of getting it can be decreased by paying attention to what you eat, drink, and touch, as well as taking preventive medication.

Before leaving on your travels and as part of the preparation for your trip, visit your physician or travel clinic to discuss measures to prevent travelers' diarrhea and how to treat it should it occur. Discuss the use of preventive medications. This type of preventive treatment is known as "prophylaxis" or taking a medication "prophylactically." If your physician or travel clinic recommends the use of antibiotics either in the prevention or the treatment of travelers' diarrhea, make sure you get a prescription for the appropriate antibiotic and fill this prescription before you set out on your travels.

➢ 1. General preventive measures

The adage "boil it, cook it, peel it, or forget it" is good advice, but very hard to adhere to. Part of the fun of travel is trying different foods, but try to follow as many of the guidelines below as possible.

Hygiene

- Wash fingers and hands frequently, especially before eating.
- Have wet wipes or antibacterial towelettes available at all times. Hand sanitizer gels are effective in killing germs on your hands.

- Always wash hands thoroughly after using the toilet.
- Try to discourage children from putting their hands and other objects into their mouths.
- If your child uses a pacifier, fasten it to your child's clothing to keep it from dropping on the floor or ground. Wash the pacifier frequently.
- Do not brush your teeth with water from fountains, streams, etc. In developing countries it may not be safe to brush your teeth with tap water.

Liquids

- Drink only safe water and beverages. Boiled water is usually the safest, but properly chemically treated water and appropriately filtered water is usually safe.
- Commercially bottled carbonated water and beverages (without ice) are usually safe. The beverage should be opened in front of you and the tops of bottles and edges of cans should be wiped clean and dry. Non-carbonated bottled water in developing countries is not necessarily safe to drink, as the bottle may have been filled at the local stream or village faucet.
- Tap water in developing countries is **not** usually safe to drink. Do **not** drink water from fountains, streams, etc.
- Do **not** add ice to a beverage unless the ice has been made from boiled water and stored in clean containers and handled in a clean fashion.
- Breastfeeding is obviously ideal for infants. If using formula, prepare the formula with bottled water, or use "ready-to-use" formula.
- For older children and adults, hot beverages such as tea and coffee are usually safe.

- Drink extra fluids if you are in a hot climate.
- **Increase liquid intake at the first sign of diarrhea.**

Foods

- Foods that are usually safe to eat:
  - Vegetables and meat that are well cooked and piping hot.
  - Fruit that needs to be peeled such as oranges and bananas. Peel the fruit yourself after washing your hands. Fruits and vegetables that do not need to be peeled should be properly washed prior to eating (see chapter on preparation of safe food and water). Wash the surfaces of fruits such as apples, oranges, and melons before cutting into them.
  - Bread and dry foods.
  - Foods with very high sugar content such as syrups and jellies are usually safe.
  - When you eat out, choose better class restaurants and hotels, although this is no guarantee that the food will not be contaminated! Avoid restaurants with many flies and poor toilet facilities.
  - Remember that when you fly home, the food that has been prepared in a developing country for the airline may be contaminated, so continue to follow these guidelines until you are back in a developed country.

FOODS AND LIQUIDS TO AVOID

- Raw and undercooked meats and fish. Avoid raw shellfish, as they may not only give you diarrhea, but also hepatitis A. (Hepatitis A can be prevented by appropriate immunization before setting out on your travels).

- Do not eat reheated foods.

- Do not eat unpasteurized dairy products, such as milk, cream, butter, or cheese. Ice cream is particularly risky.

- Avoid raw and undercooked eggs.

- Do not eat custards, salads with mayonnaise, or foods that have been allowed to stand out for some time (such as salads and buffets). Quiches and spicy sauces are ideal culture mediums for bacteria!

- Do not buy food from a street vendor unless it is fresh and steaming hot, you have watched it being prepared, and it has been handled minimally by the vendor after cooking. Particularly avoid "slushies," ice cream, fruit juices sold at fruit stands, and other similar foods that can be purchased on the street.

- Fruits and vegetables such as strawberries and lettuce are hard to wash properly and are especially risky.

- Tap water and drinks containing ice are often contaminated.

Even if you adhere to the guidelines above closely, you may still get travelers' diarrhea! This is probably because of the contamination of food during preparation, handling, and storage. Flies may also play a major part in the contamination of food.

➤ 2. Medications to _prevent_ travelers' diarrhea

As mentioned above before you set out on your travels discuss these medications with your physician or travel clinic and acquire them prior to your travels.

Pepto Bismol

Is approximately sixty percent effective in preventing travelers' diarrhea.

To prevent travelers' diarrhea, some experts believe that *Pepto Bismol* should be taken prophylactically by adults and children older than three years of age when traveling to especially high-risk countries. There are **contraindications to taking *Pepto Bismol*.** See list below.

Do Not Take *Pepto Bismol* in These Circumstances:

- Do not take *Pepto Bismol* if you have aspirin allergies, bleeding disorders, or take anticoagulant medications.
- Do not take *Pepto Bismol* if you have a history of peptic ulcer disease or gastrointestinal bleeding.
- Do not take *Pepto Bismol* if you are taking aspirin.
- *Pepto Bismol* should not be given to children who have chicken pox or a flu-like illness. See comment on Reye's syndrome.
- *Pepto Bismol* should probably **not** be given to children below three years of age.

Side Effects

- These include black stools and/or a black tongue. These side effects are medically insignificant.

- Ringing in the ears is a sign of overdosage.
- Overdoses of *Pepto Bismol* will cause the same side effects as salicylate (aspirin) poisoning and can be very serious. **Keep *Pepto Bismol* in a safe place away from the inquisitive hands of young children.**

  Pepto Bismol contains salicylates similar to the salicylates found in aspirin. There are 102 mg. of salicylates in every tablet of *Pepto Bismol* and 129 mg. of salicylates in every 1 tbsp. (15 ml.) of *Pepto Bismol* liquid. Approximately 3 *Pepto Bismol* tablets or 2½ tbsp. (1¼ oz.) contain as much as salicylate as 1 adult aspirin tablet.

- The chronic use of *Pepto Bismol* may cause constipation.

Pepto Bismol and Reye's Syndrome

Reye's syndrome has never been reported as a complication of taking *Pepto Bismol*. However, it is probably wise **not** to give *Pepto Bismol* to your child if she has chicken pox or a flu-like illness.

Pepto Bismol and Antibiotics

- *Pepto Bismol* should **not** be taken at the same time as antibiotics, as *Pepto Bismol* may interfere with the absorption of antibiotics. Wait at least two hours between doses of *Pepto Bismol* and antibiotics.

Forms of *Pepto Bismol*

Pepto Bismol is available in several forms:

1. Pleasant tasting chewable tablets, each containing 262 mg. of bismuth subsalicylate.
2. *Pepto Bismol* caplets, each containing 262 mg. of bismuth subsalicylate.
3. *Pepto Bismol* liquid—3 tsp. (1 tbsp. or ½ an ounce) of liquid contain 262 mg. of bismuth subsalicylate.

Tablets and liquids are both equally effective in the *prevention* of travelers' diarrhea. *Pepto Bismol* liquid is slightly more effective than *Pepto*

Bismol tablets in the treatment of travelers' diarrhea. The tablets are obviously more convenient than liquids when you are traveling.

PEPTO BISMOL DOSAGE FOR <u>PREVENTIVE</u> TREATMENT

Pepto Bismol is most effective if **taken with meals.** The fourth daily dose can be given at bedtime.

Children over twelve years and adults:

- 2 tablets or 2 tbsp. (1 oz.) of liquid four times a day.

Children three to twelve years:

- 1 tablet or 1 tbsp. (½ oz.) of liquid four times a day. (Many physicians believe that *Pepto Bismol* should not be given to children below six years of age.)

Children less than three years of age:

- **Not** indicated.

Antibiotics

Antibiotics are generally <u>**not**</u> **recommended as *prophylaxis*** for travelers' diarrhea for the following reasons:

- Side effects to antibiotics may occur. These include the development of yeast infections and antibiotic allergies.
- The bacteria that cause the diarrhea may develop resistance to antibiotics, which makes the treatment of travelers' diarrhea more difficult if it should occur.

- People taking preventive medications may be less likely to follow the other preventive guidelines such as choosing safe food and water and hand washing.

Antibiotics may be indicated in certain high risk individuals such as those with underlying bowel diseases or defects in immunity.

Probiotics

Probiotics such as lactobacillus have a modest effect in preventing travelers' diarrhea but cannot be relied upon on their own.

B. *TREATMENT* OF TRAVELERS' DIARRHEA

Refer also to the chapter on vomiting, diarrhea, and dehydration, page 257.

There is a wide range in the severity of travelers' diarrhea. Most people have a few loose stools a day. Other people become severely ill and pass large quantities of watery diarrhea and have severe vomiting and may become dehydrated. Fortunately, travelers' diarrhea is not usually a dehydrating illness in adolescents and adults.

Infants and younger children (below three years of age) and the elderly, are at greater risk of becoming dehydrated, but even adults may become seriously dehydrated if the diarrhea is severe enough. This is especially likely to happen if the person is also vomiting, is in a hot climate, or is not drinking enough fluid.

The younger the child and the more severe the diarrhea, the more vital it is to use ideal fluids such

as commercially prepared electrolyte solution. These should be used in the correct quantities. It is very important to observe your child carefully for signs of dehydration.

Treatment *consists* of the following:

- Fluids and nutrition.
- Medications such as *Pepto Bismol,* loperamide (*Imodium*), and antibiotics.

Treatment *depends* on the following:

- Severity of the diarrhea.
- Age of the individual.
- Presence of complicating factors such as dehydration, fever, blood and mucus in the stools (dysentery), and abdominal pain.

Caution

Under no circumstances should the administration of *Pepto Bismol, Imodium,* or antibiotics take precedence over the administration of appropriate fluids to young children with diarrhea. The most common mistake in taking care of children with diarrhea is to give them insufficient fluids. The next most common mistake is to give them inappropriate fluids such as full-strength juices, therefore making the diarrhea worse.

Fluids and Nutrition

The following treatment advice is broken down by **severity** (mild diarrhea, moderate to severe diarrhea) **within two age groups** (infants and young children, and older children and adults).

1. Follow the specific instructions for age and severity.
2. Read the section "Points to Note with Fluid and Nutritional Therapy," which follows the specifics for age and severity.

In all cases:

1. **Increase fluid intake on hot days.**
2. **Increase fluid intake at the first sign of diarrhea.**
3. **Continue giving extra fluids until the diarrhea has resolved.**

A person's activity level or energy level, as well as the urine color, are usually good guides to the presence of dehydration. For further information on assessing dehydration, refer to the table on page 260.

Infants and young children

I) Mild diarrhea in infants and young children (who are not dehydrated)

These comments apply particularly to children between the ages of six months and three years. For infants below six months of age you should consult your child's physician.

a) Fluids and nutrition
- Continue with the usual diet (breastmilk or formula) and your child's usual solids. Breastfed children should be fed more often.

- Give extra fluids between usual feeds. These fluids should consist of water, **diluted** juices (one-third strength), sports drinks such as *Gatorade* or *Jello* (both half strength). These fluids should preferably be given with the solids mentioned right below.

- Offer foods such as cooked cereal, bananas, rice, and mashed potatoes, all of which aid in the absorption of water from the intestine. Bananas are a good source of potassium.

- Children above eighteen months of age can be offered salty crackers or pretzels as a source of salt.

- If the diarrhea becomes more severe, preferably use electrolyte solutions.

- Be alert for the symptoms and signs of worsening diarrhea and dehydration!

See also chapter on "Diarrhea and Dehydration," section on "Treating Mild Illness with no Dehydration," page 261.

b) Medications
Medications are rarely indicated in such circumstances.

II) Moderate to severe diarrhea in infants and young children (less than three years)

These children are likely to have large watery stools. They may be explosive and occur every hour or even more frequently. Dehydration may occur rapidly. You will need to assess your child repeatedly for the presence of dehydration.

a) Fluids and nutrition
- If your child is dehydrated follow the guidelines in the chapter on diarrhea and dehydration. (page 257)

- **The really important aspects of this thera-py are:**
  - — Give appropriate electrolyte solutions, frequently and in sufficient amounts.
  - — Give extra fluids for each watery stool.
  - — Continue giving extra fluids until the diarrhea has resolved.
  - — Avoid fluids and foods that will make the diarrhea worse.
  - — Do not starve your child.
  - — Assess the degree of dehydration frequently.

b) Medications

- Consider giving *Imodium* if your child is over two years of age. (See "Using medications to treat travelers' diarrhea" page 121)
- Occasionally, the administration of antibiotics may be indicated (See "Using medications to treat travelers' diarrhea" page 121)

Older children and adults

I) Mild to moderate diarrhea in older children (three years and older) and adults

a) Fluids and nutrition

- Continue with the usual diet, but avoid caffeine-containing beverages and alcohol.
- Consume extra fluids in the form of water, diluted juices, and sodas (one-third strength), *Gatorade* (half strength), soup, or electrolyte solution. Give these fluids with the solids below.

- Saltine-type crackers (salted crackers), pretzels, lightly-salted cooked cereal, and mashed potatoes are a good source of extra salt if the main source of fluid is water or diluted juices. Bananas are a good source of extra potassium.

- As the severity of the diarrhea increases, increase the amount of fluid consumed. Adolescents and adults may need as much as four or more liters (four or more quarts or sixteen or more 8-oz. cups) of extra fluid in a twenty-four- hour period.

➡ **Be alert for worsening diarrhea and signs of dehydration.**

b) Medications

- Consider giving *Imodium* and antibiotics if the diarrhea is severe. (See "Using medication to treat travelers' diarrhea" page 121.)

- Reassess the situation in twenty-four hours. If the diarrhea is still profuse and watery, continue with a three day course of antibiotics and possibly *Imodium*.

II) Severe diarrhea in older children (older than three years) and adults

a) Fluids and nutrition

- Unless vomiting, continue with the usual diet, but avoid alcohol, caffeine-containing beverages, and dairy products.

- Offer large volumes of electrolyte solutions. Adolescents and adults may need to drink an extra five to six liters (five to six quarts, twenty to thirty or more 8-oz. cups) of fluid per twenty-four hours.

- Continue drinking extra fluids as long as the diarrhea continues and until the urine is a light color.
- Give additional extra fluids (up to twelve ounces) after each loose stool is passed.
- Give supplemental food as mentioned in the section for mild to moderate diarrhea above.

➲ **Observe for worsening symptoms and signs of dehydration.**

b) Medication

- Give antibiotics and possibly *Imodium* (see below, page 124).
- Reassess the situation in twenty-four hours. If the diarrhea is still significant, continue with a three day course of antibiotics and possibly *Imodium*. (For dosages and side effects of *Imodium* see below.)

Points to note with fluid and nutritional therapy

1. Concentrated liquids

- In young children **avoid** concentrated juices and full-strength *Jello, Gatorade,* and sodas. These have very high sugar content, little or no salts, and will often make the diarrhea worse.
- Diluted versions of the above fluids may be used for short periods with mild to moderate diarrhea, and

especially if supplemented with salty foods such as salted crackers or pretzels. Use one-third strength fruit juices and sodas, half strength sports drinks such as *Gatorade* and half strength *Jello*.

- Do **not** use chicken broth, because it has too much salt and no sugar, and is not suitable for rehydration in infants and young children.

- Avoid caffeine-containing drinks.

- **The younger the child and the more severe the diarrhea, the more important it is to use appropriate electrolyte solutions.** However, if you do not have commercially available electrolyte solutions or the necessary ingredients to make up homemade electrolyte solution, it is still essential to give what fluids you have available. Water, half-strength sports drinks such as *Gatorade,* half-strength *Jello,* and one-third-strength juices can be given along with saltine-type crackers.

2. Vomiting

- If your child is vomiting, stop all solids and liquids other than the clear liquid mentioned below for four to six hours.

- Offer electrolyte solutions or other clear fluids such as water, diluted juices, or sports drinks. Give as little as one teaspoon every minute. Even infants and young children who are vomiting will usually be able to tolerate **small** volumes of such fluids.

- You may need to use a teaspoon or medicine dropper in an infant.

- In older children, you may use a medicine cup. As the fluid is tolerated, increase the volumes offered. Children above eighteen months of age may suck on ice chips if vomiting is a problem. Electrolyte solutions may be made into popsicles which your child can suck, or into ice cubes, which can then be crushed and offered as ice chips.

- If your child continues to vomit, medical care should be sought.

3. Food

- If your child is vomiting, you should stop his or her normal diet for a period of four to six hours, and then try to reintroduce appropriate foods slowly.

- Do **not** starve your child. Cereal, mashed potatoes, rice, wheat, and bananas will actually aid in water absorption, shorten the period of diarrhea, and decrease its severity.

- It is usually not necessary or advisable to dilute milk or formulas unless your child is vomiting and, even then, do it for only short periods.

- Avoid fatty foods for two to three days.

Using medications to *treat* travelers' diarrhea

Caution

Under no circumstances should the administration of *Pepto Bismol*, *Imodium*, or antibiotics take precedence over the administration of appropriate fluids to young children with diarrhea.

A) *PEPTO BISMOL*

Pepto Bismol may be used in the treatment as well as the prevention of travelers' diarrhea.

See earlier section on the use of *Pepto Bismol* discussed above.

Recommended doses of *Pepto Bismol* in the <u>treatment</u> of diarrhea.

The *first* dose of *Pepto Bismol* is as follows:

Children above 12 years of age and adults:

2 tablets or 2 tbsp. (1 oz.)

Children 9 to 12 years of age:

1 tablet or 1 tbsp.

Children 6 to 9 years of age:

2 tsp.

Children 3 to 6 years of age:

1 tsp.

(Many physicians do not recommend *Pepto Bismol* for children below six years of age).

Below three years of age:

not recommended.

***Subsequent* doses:**

The above doses can be repeated every hour to a maximum of eight doses in a twenty-four- hour period.

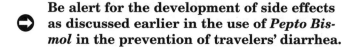

Be alert for the development of side effects as discussed earlier in the use of *Pepto Bismol* in the prevention of travelers' diarrhea.

B) LOPERAMIDE (*IMODIUM*)

Imodium reduces both the frequency of stools and the duration of diarrheal illness.

Side effects of *Imodium* include drowsiness, abdominal distension, and vomiting. **If these occur, stop the *Imodium* immediately.** If the abdominal distension persists for longer than four to six hours consult a physician.

Caution

***Imodium* should not be used if there is blood or mucus in the stools or if a high fever is present.**

Imodium is available in several forms:

1. Liquid—which contains 1 mg. of loperamide per 5 ml. (1 tsp.).
2. Chewable tablets—which contains 2 mg. of loperamide per tablet.
3. Caplets—which contains 2 mg. of loperamide per tablet.

DOSAGE OF IMODIUM IN THE *TREATMENT* OF DIARRHEA

Adults and children over twelve years

— 2 caplets or 2 tablets immediately.

— Then 1 caplet or tablet after each watery stool.

— Do not give more than 8 caplets or tablets in a twenty-four-hour period.

Children ages nine to eleven years (or between sixty and ninety-five pounds)

— 1 caplet or one chewable tablet or 2 tsp. after the first loose stool.

— then ½ caplet or ½ tablet or 1 tsp. after each subsequent loose stool.

— Do not give more than 6 tsp. or 3 caplets or tablets per twenty-four-hour period.

Children ages six to eight years (or between forty-eight and fifty-nine pounds)

— 1 caplet or 1 chewable tablet or 2 tsp. after the first loose stool.

— Then ½ caplet or ½ tablet or 1 tsp. after each subsequent loose stool.

— Do not give more than 4 tsp. or 2 caplets a day.

Children ages two to five years (or between twenty-four and forty-seven pounds)

— ½ a chewable tablet or 1 tsp. after the first loose stool.

— then ½ a chewable tablet or 1 tsp. after each subsequent loose stool.

— Do not give more than 1½ chewable tablets or 3 tsp. per day.

➡ **Use with caution in this age group.**

Below 2 years of age—*not* recommended.

Caution

Never use Diphenonxylate hydro-chloride (*Lomotil*) in the treatment of diarrhea in children.

C) ANTIBIOTICS IN THE *TREATMENT* OF DIARRHEA

Antibiotics are often very effective in the treatment of travelers' diarrhea. This is because most cases of travelers' diarrhea are due to bacteria.

The traditional approach to the treatment of travelers' diarrhea in children has been ***not*** to use antibiotics or *Imodium*. Although this may be correct in the management of childhood diarrhea which occurs at home, this may not be so in the treatment of *travelers' diarrhea*. **The combination of antibiotics and *Imodium* is usually very effective in stopping travelers' diarrhea.** Antibiotics treat the cause of the diarrhea whereas fluids prevent and treat dehydration.

Many different types of antibiotics are used in the treatment of travelers' diarrhea. Discuss this with your physician prior to traveling. The most suitable antibiotic will vary according to your destination, the season of the year, and from year to year. The age of the person taking the antibiotic may also affect the choice of the antibiotic. In 2004, azithromycin (*Zithromax*), *rifaximin*, or a quinolone antibiotic are often recommended. The antibiotics may be given as a single dose or as a three-day course.

NOTE:

The use of antibiotics in some cases of diarrhea may be dangerous, as they may precipitate a rare but serious illness known as hemolytic uremic syndrome. This may occur if the diarrhea is due to specific strains of E. coli. (Travelers' diarrhea in Argentina is sometimes caused by this strain of E. coli.) It is for this reason that many experts are loathe to recommend the use of antibiotics in children who have travelers' diarrhea, unless the specific bacterial cause of the diarrhea is known. This is one of the reasons why it is so important to discuss the treatment of travelers' diarrhea with a travel clinic or physician **before** you set out on your travels. Certainly if your child develops travelers' diarrhea **after** returning to the United States it would be prudent to test your child's stools to identify the infectious agent that is causing the diarrhea before treating with antibiotics. However, most cases of travelers' diarrhea are **not** due to these specific strains of E.coli.

DIFFERENCES BETWEEN CHILDHOOD DIARRHEA "BACK HOME" AND TRAVELERS' DIARRHEA

"Usual" Childhood Diarrhea	Travelers' Diarrhea
Usually viral	Usually bacterial
Not usually helped by using antibiotics (in fact, antibiotics usually contra-indicated)	Often helped by using antibiotics (either antibiotics alone or a combination of antibiotics and *Imodium*)
You have all the advantages of being at home (e.g. easy access to a kitchen, clean fluids, medications, and medical care.)	You have all the disadvantages of being away from home.

In both types of diarrhea it is essential to pay attention to fluid and nutritional therapy.

WHEN TO SEEK MEDICAL ATTENTION FOR TRAVELERS' DIARRHEA

Reasons to seek medical care are similar to those mentioned in the chapter on diarrhea and dehydration. Finding medical care while traveling is not always easy but the presence of any of the following features indicate you need to seek medical care.

- In an infant six months old or younger. **Generally, the younger the child, the earlier you should seek expert medical advice.**
- If your child is limp and lethargic, or appears very ill.
- If your child has moderate to severe dehydration.
- Worsening dehydration despite appropriate fluid therapy.
- Persistent vomiting.
- Your child will not take fluids by mouth.
- If your child has a stomach ache lasting longer than two hours. Note, however, that many children have recurrent bouts of abdominal pain or cramps, especially when passing gas or stools. Persisting pain (longer than one or two hours) or worsening pain indicate the need to seek medical attention to rule out more serious causes of pain such as appendicitis, bowel perforation, obstruction, etc.
- If the stool contains a large amount of mucus or blood, or is black (and your child is not taking *Pepto Bismol*).
- If the diarrhea is not *improving* after three to four days. It may take as long as seven to ten days before your child's stools are totally normal, but each day there should be improvement. Your child should be eating and drinking well, and be active, alert, and interested in his or her surroundings.
- High fever (greater than 102°F (38°C)).
- Diarrhea that continues or reoccurs after returning home.
- You should seek medical attention earlier in any country where such diseases as cholera, typhoid, or amebiasis are common, especially if such countries are having epidemics or outbreaks of these diseases.

HOMEMADE ELECTROLYTE SOLUTIONS

Here are four recipes for making your own electrolyte solutions.

Sugar and salt mixture

4 to 5 level tsp. sugar
1 **level** tsp. salt
1 quart water (approximately 1 liter)

Rice cereal mixture

1 **level** tsp. salt
1 cup (50 gm.) rice cereal
1 quart water (approximately 1 liter)

Dissolve the salt and water, gradually adding cereal to the water until the mixture is thick but still drinkable. Mix well.

Orange juice mixture

8 oz. orange juice (1 cup)
1 **level** tsp. salt
24 oz. water (3 cups)

Mashed potato mixture

8 oz. mashed potatoes
1/2 level tsp. salt
1/4 level tsp. baking soda
1/4 level tsp. salt substitute (provides potassium)
1 quart water (approximately 1 liter)

SELECTING AND PREPARING SAFE FOOD AND WATER

(See also: Section on Travelers' Diarrhea on page 102.)

One of the most important aspects of safe travel is preventing illness acquired from contaminated food and water. In the developed world, the availability of safe, drinkable water is usually taken for granted. In fact, when one stops to think about it, the ability to turn on a faucet and get abundant clear water which is safe to drink is almost a miracle and must be regarded as one of the major advances of the twentieth century! In contrast, **in many developing countries, the water is not safe to drink, even though it might come out of a faucet.** The load of infectious organisms may be high because of inadequate water treatment or outdated plumbing. **In general, all water in developing countries should be considered contaminated and capable of causing disease,** usually diarrhea. Surface water is often highly contaminated with human waste. Much of the disease, malnutrition, and shortened life span in developing countries are related to poor sanitation and contaminated water. Unsafe drinking water causes millions of deaths a year, especially in young children, where repeated bouts of diarrhea lead to malnutrition and poor health.

Even in North America, all untreated water should be considered contaminated. This includes water from mountain streams, rivers, and

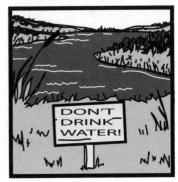

crystal clear lakes. Contrary to popular opinion, fast running, pristine mountain streams may also harbor disease-causing organisms, especially Giardia, which causes the disease giardiasis. Bloating, chronic diarrhea, and weight loss are some of the symptoms of giardiasis.

Although diarrhea and other intestinal illnesses are commonly caused by intentionally drinking water, sometimes water is unintentionally ingested while participating in recreational activities such as swimming and boating. Many children and even adults swallow large amounts of water while swimming. Outbreaks of disease due to Giardia, Shigella and hepatitis A and E and many other organisms have occurred in the United States from recreational water exposure. Infants and young children often swallow large amounts of water while taking a bath!

One does not have to drink water to acquire certain water-borne diseases. This applies particularly to a disease known as schistosomiasis in which the organism enters the body directly through the skin. This disease is particularly common in Africa and certain parts of Asia. As in the case of giardiasis, this disease may not manifest for many weeks, months or even years after acquiring it. Generally speaking, it is not even safe to wade in rivers in Africa.

People usually do not acquire infections from swimming in a sea, unless they swim in an area into which sewage flows.

Water may contain not only infectious organisms but also chemical pollutants which may be hazardous to one's health. These chemicals may come from industrial sources or runoff from farms where pesticides and fertilizers are used. Pollutants often seriously damage our environment, so it may not only be unsafe to drink the water, but also unsafe to eat the fish swimming in the water! (Sadly, we are not doing a very good job of taking care of this planet for our children and our grandchildren!)

The risks of acquiring infectious diseases from water are related to a number of factors:

a) The number of infectious particles in the water (the infectious load).

b) The virulence of the infectious organisms.

c) Human (host) factors.

People at greater risk of acquiring diseases from contaminated water include:

— young children (especially infants).

— people with certain gastrointestinal diseases such as inflammatory bowel disease (Crohn's disease or ulcerative colitis).

— people with immune defects (such as people who are on immunosuppressive drugs).

— the elderly.

— pregnant women.

For these high risk people, it is especially important to drink only safe water.

Infectious agents that may be present in water can be divided into viruses, bacteria, protozoa, and parasites. These vary greatly in size and in their ability to resist eradication.

The preparation of safe (potable) water.

The preparation of safe water is known as **disinfection.** This is not the same as sterilization, as the water may not be totally free of organisms. However, the water does not contain sufficient numbers of organisms to cause disease.

Before embarking on disinfection of the water, it is necessary to **select** the water and then to get it as **clear** as possible.

A) Selecting the water

At times, water from a faucet may not be available and you may have to rely on other sources of water. Spring water and collected rain water are likely to be cleaner than surface water, such as water from rivers, streams, and ponds. Fast-moving water is preferable to stagnant water. Similarly, clear, colorless, odorless water is probably safer than discolored water that may contain debris. When collecting water from a lake or pond, try not to disturb the bottom. Select the clearer water just below the surface. When camping, choose water upstream of human habitation.

B) Obtaining clear water

If the water is very cloudy, it is a good idea to clear the water before proceeding with further disinfection. Clarifying the water not only makes it more aesthetically pleasing but also makes further filtration or chemical treatment a lot easier. Clarification can be achieved by:

1. Sedimentation. Allow the water to stand for several hours and pour off the clean upper portion for further treatment.
2. Filtration. Filter the water through a commercial paper filter, a coffee filter, or a clean cloth.
3. Flocculation. Get the organic impurities to clump together by adding a pinch of alum to the water and mixing.

C) Disinfecting the water

There are three commonly used methods to disinfect water:

1. Heat treatment
2. Chemical treatment
3. Filtration

Each of these methods may be used alone or in combination with another method. The method you choose depends on a number of factors, including the type of organism you wish to eradicate, the amount of water you need to prepare, and the resources available. A full discussion of this is beyond the scope of this book. For further information, consult the references listed at the end of this chapter. If you are planning a prolonged stay in a developing country or traveling in the wilderness, it would definitely be a good idea to do further reading on the subject.

1. **Heat treatment.**
   a) **Boiling water**
      - **Boiling water is the most reliable way to purify water.** However, it is not always feasible to do this, as a source of electricity or other fuel is necessary. If you are staying in hotels, all you may need is a small electrical heating coil or a portable kettle. Remember that the electrical current and electrical outlets in many countries differ from those in the United States. It is a good idea to take a selection of electrical outlet adapters with you.

      - **It is necessary to only bring the water to a boil to kill all offending organisms.** For an extra margin of safety you can let the water boil for one minute, or alternatively, keep the water covered so that it retains its heat for a longer time.

   b) **Pasteurization**
      Microorganisms vary in their heat sensitivity. It is not necessary to bring water to the boil to kill most bacteria and viruses. Most bacteria and viruses are killed at much lower temperatures (60–70° centigrade) as long as they are exposed

to heat for longer periods (thirty minutes or longer). This is the principle of pasteurization. In practice, when you are traveling and you don't have a means of checking the water temperature, it is usually easier just to bring the water to the boil. It is also much safer, as some organisms are more resistant to heat.

c) Hot tap water

If you have no other means of disinfecting water, then hot tap water is probably the safest. There will be far fewer organisms in hot tap water than in cold tap water, but the safety of the water cannot be guaranteed.

Generally, in most countries, it is safe to use water from a tap to clean your teeth. Although the water may contain organisms, you are unlikely to ingest a sufficient number to cause disease. However, **the high risk groups mentioned above, especially young children should only use totally safe water.**

Water that is boiled often has a rather flat taste. You can **improve the taste of treated water** as follows:

- Add a vitamin C tablet or vitamin C powder to the water and shake.
- Pour the water from one clean container into another back and forth to aerate it.
- Allow the water to stand for a while in a clean, partially filled container.
- Pass the water through a charcoal filter.

2. Chemical treatment of water

The chemical disinfection of water is usually accomplished by adding one of the following:

a) Chlorine dioxide

b) Chlorine

c) Iodine

Many different preparations of the above three chemical agents are available. Follow the directions on the bottle. Be aware of expiration dates.

The efficacy of the various methods of chemical disinfection is affected by many factors, but especially by: the concentration of the chemical agent; the turbidity of the water; the temperature of the water.

a) **Chlorine Dioxide**

Chlorine dioxide is a fairly recently marketed method of water disinfection. It is marketed in the United States, under the trade names *Pristine* and *Aquamira*. It uses a quick and easy two-step process that renders the water completely safe without the disadvantages of the unpleasant taste imparted to the water by chlorine or iodine discussed below. This method of water disinfection is highly recommended.

b) **Chlorine**

The chlorine is added to the water and left to stand for thirty minutes. If the water is cold or cloudy, either double the recommended dose of chlorine or double the contact time. Two chlorine formulations are commonly used—chlorine bleach and chlorine tablets.

Chlorine bleach: Ordinary household bleach (*Clorox*), a 4–6 % solution may be used. Add two to three drops of chlorine bleach to each litre (quart) of water.

Chlorine tablets: These are commonly marketed as *Halozone* tablets. Add two tablets to one litre (quart) of water.

Chlorine may *not* kill all organisms, especially Cryptosporidium and Cyclospora. Giardia cysts are also relatively resistant to chlorine. Chlorine may also impart a rather unpleasant taste to the water. The taste can be improved by adding a vitamin C tablet or powder to the water or passing it through a charcoal filter.

c) Iodine

Add the iodine to the water and allow it to stand for thirty minutes. If the water is cold or cloudy either double the recommended dose of iodine or double the contact time. Several forms of iodine are available to disinfect water. Iodine is light sensitive and should be stored in a dark bottle.

Iodine solutions: These include tincture of iodine (2%) and *Lugol's* solution (5%). If using tincture of iodine, add five drops to one liter (quart) of water. If using *Lugol's* iodine, add two to three drops to one litre (quart) of water.

Iodine tablets (Tetraglycine hydroperiodide): The best known preparation is sold as *Potable Aqua*. Add half a tablet to one litre (quart) of water.

As with chlorine, iodine may not kill all organisms (notably Cryptosporidium and Cyclospora) and also imparts an unpleasant taste to the water which can be improved by adding a vitamin C tablet or by passing the water through a granular activated charcoal filter.

Caution

- **Do not use iodine preparations for longer than one month, and do not use if you are pregnant.**
- **Do not use iodine if you have thyroid disease.**
- **Do not use if you are allergic to iodine.**

If there is concern that Cyclospora or Cryptosporidium may be present in the water, then the water should be filtered either before or after chemical treatment. Cryptosporium and Cyclospora may both be present in water in the wilderness in the United States.

3. Filtration

Filtration is another commonly used method of water disinfection. Be skeptical of claims made by manufacturers that their filtering devices render the water "completely safe." **The principle disadvantage of filtration is that it does not remove viruses, the smallest infectious particles.** Filtration, especially if the pore size is no larger than 0.2 to 1.0 μm, will remove bacteria, parasites and cysts but not viruses. Another disadvantage of filtering systems is that they often are bulky and tend to clog.

Filters made of porcelain (ceramic candles) that are commonly purchased in developing countries are **not** reliable.

More details on filters and filtration can be found in the references at the end of the chapter.

NOTES:

- If you are in a location where it is likely that disease-causing viruses may be in the water and filtration is used as the method of disinfection, then you must use another method besides filtration to destroy viruses. This would be the case if you were using surface water in developing countries where there is a high likelihood of contamination of the water by human fecal organisms. You should then either boil the water or use one of the chemical methods mentioned above.

- In some situations, viruses may not be a problem and filtration on its own may suffice. An example of such a situation is in the remote wilderness where there is minimal likelihood of contamination from human fecal material and the primary concern is ridding the water of Giardia and other large organisms.

The bottom line is that to obtain completely safe water, you must either drink water that has been boiled or water that has been filtered and then chemically treated. The filtration will remove the larger organisms and the chemical treatment will kill viruses.

If water is stored for a time, it should be covered and an appropriate dose of a chemical disinfectant added to prevent contamination.

Additional reminders and comments.

- In developing countries even water that comes in sealed bottles may not be safe to drink. Carbonated water is generally safer. It is preferable for the bottles to be opened in front of you.

- Unless ice is made from safe water and handled in a clean fashion, it should be regarded as contaminated.

- **Water safety cannot be assessed by look, smell, or taste.** Even pristine surface waters may contain Giardia cysts and other organisms. Remote lakes and streams that contain crystal clear water may be contaminated by disease-causing organisms.

- Chemical hazards are becoming an increasing problem and will not be removed by boiling or other methods of disinfection.

- Be sensitive to the local population who may not have access to clean food and water as you do.

Preparation of clean food.

- **Remember, most cases of travelers' diarrhea are acquired from eating contaminated food and <u>not</u> from drinking contaminated water.**

- **Foods to avoid:**
  - — Unpasteurized dairy products.
  - — Undercooked meats and fish.
  - — Reheated foods.
  - — Lettuce and other leafy vegetables which are difficult to wash. These are often fertilized with human waste in developing countries. (See section on travelers' diarrhea.)

- If you intend to eat fruit and vegetables that do not need to be peeled, clean them in one of the following ways:
  - — Wash them thoroughly in clean, soapy water, and then rinse them in disinfected (treated) water. (Just rinsing the fruits and vegetables in treated water may not be sufficient because it does not allow enough contact time for the chemical to kill any disease-causing organisms.)
  - — Soak fruits and vegetables in treated water that has two to three times the concentration of iodine or chlorine than is recommended for water disinfection.
  - — Dip the food in boiling water.

- **Plates, cups, glasses, and eating utensils** should also be washed in a clean fashion. This can either be achieved by washing them in boiling water or by washing them in a very strong chemical solution, again using a solution two to three times stronger than that recommended for water disinfection.

- **Storage.** Water, food, and eating utensils, once cleaned, should be stored properly so that they are not contaminated by flies which may carry disease-causing organisms.

- **Remember to wash your hands well before and after handling the food.**

Non-infections diseases that can be acquired from eating food and drinking beverages.

Although most illnesses acquired from drinking water or eating food are infectious in nature, some are due to **toxins,** and these will not be affected by the disinfection methods described.

Staphylococcal food poisoning usually presents with severe nausea and vomiting, two to six hours after eating contaminated food. High-risk foods include creamy desserts, salads, and meats, especially if they are not eaten soon after preparation.

Fish and shellfish poisoning. Shellfish may contain toxins when they feed on certain algae that proliferate during the warmer months ("red tide"). Many tropical fish contain toxins that can cause severe illness, paralysis, and even death. Even commonly eaten fish such as red snapper and grouper may be unsafe to eat if they are caught at certain times of the year. A discussion on this topic is beyond the scope of this book, but you should always be cautious when eating seafood.

Most of the toxins found in fish and shellfish are *not* destroyed by ordinary cooking. **Foods and seafood that are contaminated by toxins or toxin-producing bacteria are difficult to recognize by appearance, odor,**

or taste. Avoid eating the skin and organs of fish. If you want to eat seafood, eat it only at top restaurants or restaurants that specialize in fresh seafood.

Chemicals, toxins, and heavy metals such as mercury are *not* removed by the disinfection processes described above. Select your water carefully. Be aware of industrial pollutants, fertilizer run-off from farmlands, and other toxic wastes. Passing the water through a charcoal filter may not only improve the taste but also rid the water of some of these substances.

Sources for further information:

1. *Wilderness Medicine,* Fourth Edition, 2001, by Paul S. Auerbach (Mosby Publishers).
2. *Water Disinfection for International and Wilderness Travels,* by Howard Backer. Clinics in infectious diseases, 2002. 34, pg 355–364.
3. *The Backpacker's Field Manual,* 1998, by Rick Curtis (Three Rivers Press).

MALARIA PREVENTION

See also section on protecting your child against insects and ticks, page 312.

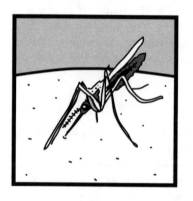

Malaria is a parasitic disease that kills almost three million people annually (mainly children) and is transmitted by the bite of the anopheles mosquito.

North Americans are particularly susceptible when traveling to malarial areas because they have never been exposed to malaria and therefore lack immunity to the malaria parasite.

If you intend to travel to an area where malaria is prevalent it is **essential** to get advice on how to prevent malaria. If you intend to spend some months in a malarial area and especially if you do not have easy access to medical care, it may be important to get guidelines on the self-diagnosis and self-treatment of malaria.

Getting advice on malaria prevention.

The prevention of malaria is extremely complex. Recommendations vary according to:

- The country you plan to visit.
- How long you intend to stay there.
- The location within the country (large cities versus rural areas, high altitude areas versus low altitude areas).

- The time of year you intend visiting the country. Many countries have a malarial season.
- The type of malaria that occurs in that country.
- The resistance pattern of the malaria parasite (this changes constantly).
- Individual factors, especially the age and the health of the person traveling to the malarial area.

For the reasons just listed, it is **strongly recommended that you visit a travel clinic** prior to your travels to discuss these issues. The physician in the clinic will assess **your risk** of malaria. Do this several weeks **before** you depart, as some anti-malarial medications need to be started at least one week before entering the malarial area. This will also give you and your physician an opportunity to assess any untoward side effects of the medication.

Detailed recommendations for the prevention of malaria can be obtained from the following sources:

1. Center for Disease Control (CDC)
   Voice Information Service: (888) 232-3228
   Fax Information Service: (888) 232-3299
   Website: http://www.cdc.gov
2. World Health Organization (WHO)
   Website: http://www.who.org
3. Shoreland's Travel Health (800) 433-5256

Malaria prevention involves two components: avoiding mosquito bites and taking anti-malarial medication:

A) *Preventing mosquito bites*

The single most important strategy in the prevention of malaria is to prevent mosquito bites. Guidelines are as follows:

Choose your destination wisely, especially if you have young children

- Within a country, certain areas have a higher malaria risk. Consider the following factors:
  - **Altitude.** High altitudes (above 1,000 meters) rarely have falciparum malaria (the worst type of malaria). This may change with global warming.
  - **Cities versus rural areas.** Malaria is less likely to be contracted in a large city than in a rural area.
  - **Seasons.** Traveling in the dry season is usually safer than traveling in or just after the rainy season.

If chloroquine-resistant malaria is present, reconsider your plans, especially if you have young children.

Clothing, perfumes and scented toiletries

- Wear clothes that cover as much of your body as possible—long pants, long-sleeved shirts, etc.
- Light-colored clothing, such as khaki, is better than dark clothing.
- Clothes can be impregnated with permethrin for added protection. This will not harm you or your child and will greatly help in deterring mosquitoes.
- Avoid using perfumes, scented soaps, and scented deodorants, which tend to attract mosquitoes.

Insect repellents

- Use an appropriate insect repellent. Preparations containing DEET are the best. Reapply as necessary. (**See section on prevention of insect bites, page 312.**)

Accommodation

- Select accommodations that have screened porches and screened windows.
- Sleep under mosquito nets. Infants and toddlers should definitely sleep in beds and cribs covered with permethrin-impregnated nets. Inspect mosquito nets for holes. If you detect any holes, repair them with thread or adhesive tape.
- Use a knock-down insecticide spray containing pyrethrin (such as *Raid* or *Doom*) in living and sleeping areas. Before retiring at night, inspect the walls and ceiling of your bedroom and kill any visible mosquitoes.
- Use an electric fan (if available) to keep the air moving. Moving air is an added deterrent to mosquitoes.

Activities

Be outdoors as little as possible from dusk to dawn—the anopheles mosquito feeds almost exclusively during these times.

B) *Anti-malarial medications*

- The next step in preventing malaria is to take appropriate anti-malarial medication. This medication does not prevent mosquito bites, nor does it prevent you from acquiring the malaria parasite.

- These medications work by preventing the later symptoms of malaria but **none** are one hundred percent effective.
- Some anti-malarial medication needs to be started one week **before** departing from home and **continued for some weeks after returning.**
- Do not skip any doses of your anti-malarial medication.
- Not all prophylactic medication may be administered to young children and infants. As mentioned before, you may have to avoid travel to a chloroquine-resistant malarial area if you are traveling with young children (most of the deaths from malaria occur in children below five years of age).
- It is also important to be aware that anti-malarial medication is extremely toxic if overdosed. Keep medication in a safe place away from the inquisitive hands of infants and young children. Take syrup of ipecac along with you in case of accidental chloroquine ingestion, as timely administration of this may literally be lifesaving.
- Remember, taking anti-malarial medication does **not** guarantee you will not get malaria.

A full discussion of anti-malarial medication is beyond the scope of this book. Further information should be obtained from your travel clinic or travel physician. It is especially important for your doctor to know whether chloroquine-resistant falciparum malaria exists and to prescribe the prophylactic medication accordingly.

Fevers and illness while in or after leaving a malarial area.

- The incubation period for malaria is at least seven days, so any illness in the first six days of travel to a malarial area is unlikely to be due to malaria.
- Because most travelers do not spend many weeks in a malarial area, the symptoms usually present once they have returned home. Malaria may take many months to manifest.
- Any unexplained fever should be taken seriously. Until proven otherwise, it should be assumed to be due to malaria. Seek expert medical help.
- If you or your children become ill while traveling in a malarial area, or on returning home from such a journey, seek medical care immediately. Inform your physician that you have been in a malarial area. **Insist** on blood tests for malaria. If these tests are negative and you remain ill, insist that these blood tests be repeated. Ask to be referred to an infectious disease specialist if your symptoms persist.

The anopheles mosquito is the most dangerous animal in Africa and is responsible for more deaths than lions, leopards, crocodiles, and other wild beasts! Do **not** underestimate the problem of malaria, especially in parts of Africa and Asia and especially in chloroquine-resistant malarial areas. **Malaria may be fatal!**

SKIN PROBLEMS WHEN TRAVELING

See also:

Section on sunburn, page 299.

Section on common skin diseases, page 148.

Section on poison ivy dermatitis, page 324.

Section on prevention of insect and tick bites, page 312.

Section on foreign adoption, page 182.

Skin problems are common and are one of the more frequent reasons travelers seek medical care both while away and after returning home. Skin problems are even more common when traveling in hot and humid environments. Most of these problems are relatively minor but can be extremely irritating and detract from the pleasure of the trip. These skin diseases range from common problems such as insect bites and sunburn to exotic parasitic diseases rarely seen in developed countries. Many of the skin diseases encountered while traveling can be prevented by **sensible sun precautions, good hygiene,** and **prevention of insect bites.** Pre-existing skin conditions may be exacerbated by the stresses of travel or by exposure to the sun.

Sunburn is the most important travel-related skin problem and is discussed separately. Insect and bug bites and their complications come a close second and these are also discussed elsewhere.

1. Heat rash/prickly heat.

This consists of a fine pimply rash which is caused by the blockage of sweat ducts. The surrounding skin becomes red so the appearance is that of small pimples surrounded by inflamed skin. As you would expect, prickly heat is more common in hot climates! This rash frequently occurs on the back and chest but it also occurs in areas where there is poor ventilation such as the arm pits and the groin and in areas where there is friction from clothing. The neck creases of infants are another common site.

Prevention:

- Dress your child in cool, loose-fitting, cotton clothing.
- Avoid friction from clothing, for example, baseball caps rubbing against the forehead.
- Bathe daily.
- Some people are more prone to prickly heat. These individuals should, if possible, spend more time in a cool or air conditioned environment.

Treatment:

- Follow the preventative measures discussed above.
- The following measures may relieve the itch and calm the rash:
  - Cool showers and Aveeno baths. Antibacterial soaps often help but tend to dry the skin.
  - Apply calamine lotion.
  - Keep the skin well aerated.
  - Try to avoid scratching the skin. Scratching may lead to impetigo.

2. Folliculitis.

Folliculitis or infection of the hair follicles often appears as clusters of bumps or little pimples. These may occur on any part of the body, but especially the buttocks, inner thighs, scalp and face. Folliculitis also is common where the scalp comes in contact with a headband or hat, where the buttocks come in contact with a sweaty, dirty seat, or where clothing rubs against the body. It is more likely to develop in hot and humid climates and with excessive sweating.

Prevention
See prevention of prickly heat above.

Treatment
See treatment of prickly heat above. Keep the skin clean and dry. Antibacterial soaps may be helpful and so may the application of antibacterial creams or ointments. For severe folliculitis, oral antibiotics may be needed.

Occasionally, folliculitis may develop into small painful boils. These may respond to hot compresses. If the boils increase in size, then lancing of the boils and oral antibiotics may be needed.

A specific type of folliculitis, known as "hot tub folliculitis," may be acquired from bathing in hot tubs or whirlpools that are not adequately chlorinated. This condition usually resolves without treatment over seven to fourteen days. (Treatment is directed at the hot tub! Make sure the hot tub water is adequately chlorinated.)

3. Impetigo.

Impetigo is the name given to a common bacterial infection of the skin. It is contagious and is caused by bacteria called streptococci (strep) or staphylococci (staph). It can be spread to other parts of the body by scratching and can also be spread to other people.

Impetigo often follows the scratching of bug bites and also occurs in areas where the skin has been broken, for example around minor cuts and abrasions. It is especially common around the nose.

Impetigo usually starts as flat reddened areas which develop into small vesicles (little blisters). These blisters rupture and discharge a yellowish fluid which dries into honey-colored crusts. The surrounding skin is red. Red satellite lesions may develop wherever the skin is scratched.

In third world countries, many children have persistent impetigo due to poor hygiene, heat, humidity, and scratching. Even in developed countries, impetigo is common and may recur frequently.

Prevention of impetigo

- Prevent insect bites. (See section on prevention of insect bites.)

- Good hygiene is very important. Frequent baths or showers will keep the bacterial population of the skin in check, especially if an antibacterial soap is used. Prevent the skin from drying out by applying a moisturizer afterwards.

- Keep as cool as possible—wear loose-fitting, cotton clothing.

- Wash and dry abrasions and cuts and keep clean. Apply an antibacterial ointment to cuts and abrasions three times a day until the skin heals. Don't cover minor bites and scratches with band-aids as this will encourage infection. Rather allow these lesions to air out and dry out. If you do cover a cut or an abrasion with a bandage or dressing, change the dressing at least once a day and allow the wound to air.

- Don't scratch bug bites. Unless the skin is broken, apply topical ½% or 1% hydrocortisone cream to the bug bite to decrease the itch and inflammation. Use an oral medication such as *Benadryl* or one of the non-sedating antihistamines to decrease the itch.

Treatment of impetigo

- Use an antibacterial cream or ointment on the lesion (examples of these are *Bacitracin, Neosporin, Triple antibiotic, Bactroban.*)
- If your child has many lesions, an antibiotic by mouth is recommended.
- For **recurring** impetigo the following may be helpful:
  — Apply *Bactroban* to the inside of the nose, three times a day for seven to ten days. Staph and strep are often harbored in the nose.
  — Bathe your child once or twice a week in a tub of water to which half a cup of bleach has been added. This will tend to dry out the skin, so apply a moisturizer afterwards. Keep the bleach in a safe place!
  — An appropriate antibiotic by mouth is often necessary. If your child is prone to impetigo and you are planning travels to a hot and humid country, it may be a good idea to request an antibiotic that you can use to treat this condition should it develop.

4. Fungal infections.

Fungal infections are particularly common in tropical and subtropical areas but occur worldwide. The more common fungal infections are athlete's foot, ringworm, yeast vaginal infections, and diaper rashes in babies. Fungi like moist, dark areas such as under the diaper and between the toes. Vaginal yeast infections are particularly common in women who are taking antibiotics. When taking an antibiotic, your likelihood of developing vaginitis (and diarrhea) can be reduced by consuming yogurt that has a live culture.

Yeast diaper rashes often appear as a bright red rash in the diaper area with surrounding satellite red spots.

This rash responds to airing the affected area, keeping it clean and dry and applying an anti-fungal cream such as clotrimazole (*Lotrimin*). Prevention of **diaper rashes** includes changing your child as soon as he is wet or dirty, keeping buttocks clean and dry and avoiding plastic, waterproof pants. See section on diaper rashes.

Athlete's Foot is the most common fungal infection seen in adolescents and adults and usually presents as an itchy, red rash between the toes. It may be **prevented** by:

— Keeping feet clean and dry.

— Changing socks frequently.

— Airing shoes at night.

— Alternating between two pairs of shoes.

— Wearing sandals instead of closed shoes and boots.

— Sprinkling an antifungal powder into shoes and socks.

— Wearing slippers or shower shoes in public places such as gyms and swimming pool showers.

Treatment of athlete's foot consists of employing the preventative measures listed above as well as the application of an antifungal cream or powder. It usually responds well to clotrimazole (*Lotrimin*) cream, terbinafine (*Lamisil*) cream or an antifungal foot powder such as tolnaftate (*Tinactin*).

NOTE: Do **not** set out on a hiking trip or vacation to tropical or subtropical climates without first taking care of athlete's foot! If you do, the heat and sweating will dramatically worsen the condition.

Ringworm is a fungal infection of the skin and is commonly spread between children and from pets to children. The lesions usually have a round or oblong shape, a clear center and a scaly advancing edge. Treatment consists of the application of antifungal creams or ointments for many weeks. Ringworm and eczema (atopic dermatitis) often look alike. They are both very common but their treatment is very different!

5. Poison ivy and contact dermatitis

These are discussed at greater length in the section on summer woes.

Many people who react to poison ivy also react to mangos, especially to mango peel and may develop a rash after eating and handling mangos.

Contact dermatitis may be due to cosmetics, suntan lotion, bracelets, watch straps, and earrings, etc. Vacationers purchase new jewelry or apply unfamiliar creams, lotions, and cosmetics, which may lead to irritant rashes. Contact dermatitis responds to steroid creams and the removal of the irritant.

6. Hives

See section on common skin disease in children.

7. Eczema/atopic dermatitis

See section on atopic dermatitis (eczema).

Eczema often gets worse during periods of travel, especially when traveling in hot and humid areas or in very cold and dry climates. Just the stresses of traveling may worsen the eczema. Prior to travel discuss with your child's doctor what you should do if your child's eczema becomes more troublesome while away. Take along a supply of medications to treat worsening eczema. This should include:

— More potent steroid creams or ointments.

— A course of oral steroids.
— A course of antibiotics appropriate for treating staph and strep infections.

Ask your doctor for an eczema action plan which sets out steps you can take to treat worsening eczema.

8. An ill child with a rash that appears suddenly and spreads rapidly.

If your child develops a rash that does not blanch (whiten) when pressure is applied to it, and which spreads rapidly, and your child is ill (e.g. has a fever and is lethargic), you should take this very seriously. This may indicate a disease called meningococcemia which may be fatal if not treated promptly. This disease occurs throughout the world, but particularly in sub-Saharan Africa and requires immediate antibacterial treatment. Some of the more serious viral infections, such as dengue fever, may also cause reddish rashes that are scattered over the entire body. **If anyone in your party is ill, has a high fever and a rash, medical care should be sought.**

NOTE:

As discussed at the beginning of this section, there are many other less common rashes that can be acquired when traveling. Bathing in tropical waters can result in painful rashes due to contact with marine creatures. Spider and insect bites may cause a variety of rashes. Physicians that work in western, more developed countries may have difficulty diagnosing some of the less common and more exotic rashes that may be acquired in tropical climates. It may be necessary to consult a dermatologist or tropical disease specialist to diagnose and treat these rashes.

- **Steroid creams and rashes.**

  — Steroid creams help to decrease the itch associated with insect bites, contact dermatitis and eczema.

  — If the skin becomes infected, these creams may encourage spread of the infection. Yeast infections also spread more rapidly when steroid creams are applied to them. Ringworm may initially appear to respond to a steroid cream but later the rash increases in size.

  — Application of steroid creams may also make subsequent diagnosis of the skin disorder far more difficult.

  — **Never** apply steroid preparations to the eyelids. Do not use strong steroid preparations on the face or underneath the diaper unless directed to do so by a physician.

ALTITUDE SICKNESS

Few of us will climb Mount Everest or Mount Kilimanjaro, but if you decide to leave the sun and warmth of the beach and fly to Aspen to ski, your body will notice the difference. You will definitely be aware of the effects of altitude if you fly into Cuzco in Peru from sea level or ascend to the top of Pike's Peak in Colorado.

What is it?

Altitude sickness is the term used to describe a spectrum of symptoms and syndromes that occur at high altitudes. All the tissues of the body are affected by the lack of oxygen at high altitude but the two organs most strikingly involved are the brain and the lungs. The milder manifestations are known as acute mountain sickness. The more severe brain manifestations are 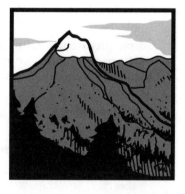 caused by brain swelling which is known as high altitude cerebral edema (HACE). The lungs may become very congested and drown in fluid and this is known as high altitude pulmonary edema (HAPE). HACE and HAPE may be fatal unless immediate measures are taken to treat them.

The terminology relating to altitude sickness is very confusing: some authors use the term "acute mountain sickness" synonymously with the term "altitude sickness" to include the entire spectrum of symptoms and syndromes from the milder manifestations to HACE and HAPE. Other authors use the term "acute mountain sickness" to include only the milder manifestations of altitude sickness.

Why does it occur?

Altitude sickness occurs when one ascends to high altitudes, especially if this is done rapidly. At high altitudes, less oxygen is available to the body. The lungs and heart have to work a lot harder to supply the muscles and the other tissues with enough oxygen to function.

Who gets it?

- **Anyone can get altitude sickness.**
- Altitude sickness is just as likely to occur in children as in adults.
- **Being physically fit at sea level does not prevent altitude sickness.** Even the most athletic teenagers and young adults who are in superb physical condition can develop fatal altitude sickness!

The likelihood of developing altitude sickness and its severity are related to:

— The altitude—the higher you go, the greater the risk.

— The speed of ascent—the faster you ascend, the greater the risk. In other words, the less time you take to acclimatize, the greater the risk.

— Physical exertion—the more you exert yourself at high altitude, the greater the risk.

— Genetic factors—some individuals are more susceptible to developing altitude sickness than others.

— You're **more** likely to get altitude sickness if you:

  • have had altitude sickness in the past.

  • are dehydrated.

- are hypothermic (have a low body temperature).
- have an infection such as an upper respiratory tract infection (URI).
- usually reside at a low altitude.
- have certain medical conditions such as chronic lung disease and some types of heart disease.

— You are **less** likely to get altitude sickness if you:

- ascend slowly and take time to acclimatize.
- keep well hydrated.
- eat a high carbohydrate diet.

At what altitudes does altitude sickness occur?

This is related to numerous factors, some of which have been mentioned above:

- Minor manifestations of altitude sickness, those seen in acute mountain sickness, are common with rapid ascent to 8,000 feet. This is the altitude at which many ski resorts are situated. Rarely, acute mountain sickness occurs at lower altitudes. The altitude at which you sleep is most important.

- Fortunately, the more serious forms of altitude illness, HACE and HAPE (described above) are uncommon below 10,000 feet. However, individual susceptibility varies and deaths have occurred at lower altitudes.

The higher you go, the greater the risk, especially if you rapidly ascend from sea level to high altitudes.

What is normal at high altitude?

- All of us get breathless with exertion at high altitude. We may also feel light-headed.
- Virtually everyone develops a cough if they ascend high enough.
- You may not sleep as well at night.
- You may have periodic breathing. This consists of cycles of breathing at a normal rate, then holding one's breath for up to ten to fifteen seconds, and then breathing rapidly.
- Increased urination is also common. This may be another cause for waking frequently at night.
- Swelling of the hands, feet, and face may occur. This is more common in women.

How do you recognize it?

Symptoms of altitude sickness usually begin within six to twelve hours of ascending to high altitude and increase in severity over the next one to two days. They are usually worse at night.

Acute Mountain Sickness

You fulfill the criteria for acute mountain sickness if you have recently ascended to a high altitude (above 8,000 feet) and have a headache as well as one of the symptoms described below:

- Nausea, vomiting, and a decrease in appetite.
- Fatigue.
- Dizziness.

- Insomnia.
- Irritability.

Adults who have had a hangover in the past will tell you acute mountain sickness is very similar.

Headache: This tends to be severe, throbbing, and located either at the front or the back of the head. It is often worse at night or early morning when awakening and is aggravated by bending over. This headache may initially respond to the administration of analgesics such as ibuprofen. As the severity of acute mountain sickness worsens, these drugs are less effective. The headache typically responds to the administration of oxygen or descent in altitude or specific medications for acute mountain sickness.

As altitude sickness increases in severity, other more alarming symptoms may emerge:

High altitude cerebral edema (HACE)

Symptoms that indicate the presence of brain swelling (HACE) are:

- Headache that does not respond to analgesics. This is serious!
- Confusion.
- Disturbances of gait (ataxia)—walking as though drunk.
- Poor coordination.
- A complete lack of motivation.
- Poor judgment. A person with HACE tends to have poor judgment, irrational behavior, and frequently denies that there is anything wrong with him! If treatment is not instituted, he may become stuporous and eventually lapse into coma.

High altitude pulmonary edema (HAPE)

Symptoms that suggest lung congestion (HAPE) are:

- **Cough** that is accompanied by **extreme fatigue** and **shortness of breath at rest.** Much later the cough may produce phlegm that is pink and frothy.

- Although **shortness of breath** with exertion occurs in almost everybody at high altitude, breathlessness should disappear fairly rapidly with rest. **If you are short of breath at rest, this is cause for concern.**

HAPE often occurs suddenly at night and may or may not be associated with symptoms of acute mountain sickness or HACE.

Altitude sickness in young children.

- It is always more difficult to diagnose any illness in very young children as they cannot vocalize their symptoms.

- Children of this age are often fussy anyway (especially if their routine is altered) and more likely to get upper respiratory infections and dehydration.

- It is difficult to detect the early signs of acute mountain sickness in children, especially in young children. Symptoms may include:

  — Excessive irritability and crying.

  — A loss of appetite.

  — Nausea and vomiting.

  — Inability to sleep.

If your child has any one of these symptoms, he should be considered to have altitude sickness and be treated accordingly.

It is probably not a good idea to travel to high altitudes (certainly above 12,000 feet) with very young children!

Other illnesses and altitude sickness

- As mentioned above, upper respiratory tract infections, hypothermia, and dehydration all increase your chances of getting altitude sickness.
- Children with asthma do **not** have any higher risk of developing altitude sickness. There may however, be other triggers that bring on an asthma attack. These include colds, cold air, and air pollution. Asthmatics traveling to Mexico City are more likely to be affected by the air pollution than the altitude! **It is unwise for asthmatics to ascend to high altitude if their asthma is not well controlled.** It is not wise for asthmatics to stray far from medical care if their asthma is poorly controlled, regardless of altitude.
- Children with severe lung diseases such as cystic fibrosis should not travel to high altitudes before being assessed by a pulmonologist (lung specialist).
- Children with Down's syndrome are more prone to altitude sickness.
- People with **sickle cell disease** will almost certainly have problems at high altitudes.
- If your child has a heart murmur, he should be evaluated by a cardiologist before traveling to high altitudes, as certain cardiac conditions predispose one to high altitude sickness.

Prevention of altitude sickness.

As always, prevention is better than cure.

- If you intend to vacation at a high altitude, you should discuss this with your physician and your child's physician. A variety of prescription medications may help you in preventing and treating high altitude sickness.

- If you are planning a vacation at these altitudes, you should make sure that the resort you are staying at is equipped to deal with acute mountain sickness.

- If you are planning to trek or climb at altitudes higher than 11,500 feet, you need to learn a lot more about the prevention and treatment of altitude sickness than is discussed here. You should have a guide with you who is experienced at recognizing and treating altitude sickness.

- **The most effective preventive measure is acclimatization.** Plan a two- to three-day stay at lower altitudes and **gradually** ascend to higher elevations. For example, if you are planning to stay at a mountain resort at an altitude of 9,000 feet, it would be advisable to stay for two to three-days at an intermediate altitude of 6,000 to 7,000 feet. However, this is not always possible if you reside at sea level and just plan the occasional skiing weekend in the mountains.

- An important dictum when climbing at high altitude is to **"climb high, sleep low."** In other words, you may make daytime exertions to high altitudes but should return to a lower altitude to sleep. **Altitude sickness tends to be worse at night when sleeping.**

- Keep well-hydrated. In other words, drink plenty of fluids.

- Eat foods high in carbohydrates.

- Avoid alcohol.

- Avoid sleeping tablets and other sedatives.
- A variety of medications may help you prevent and treat altitude sickness. These include acetazolomide (*Diamox*) and steroids. *Diamox* accelerates acclimatization. Prophylactic *Diamox* is an especially good idea for those skiing weekends at high altitude when you don't have time to acclimatize.

CAUTION

- You should not take Diamox if you are allergic to sulpha medication.
- Medications such as Diamox may decrease your risk of altitude sickness but not totally prevent it.

A further discussion of medications to prevent and treat altitude sickness is beyond the scope of this book.

How to treat Altitude Sickness

Treatment of altitude sickness depends on its severity. **Descent will treat all forms of altitude sickness.**

Early recognition is vital.

If you or your child has developed any of the symptoms of altitude sickness, then you should assume you have altitude sickness and consider descent to a lower altitude. Certainly ascend no further.

Never leave someone with altitude sickness alone!

Acute mountain sickness with mild symptoms:

- **Do not ascend any further! Do not ascend any further!**
- Rest, drink fluids, and take medications for headache and altitude sickness. You should rest at the same altitude for a day or two.
- **If the symptoms persist, descend.** It is often only necessary to descend 1,000 feet or so to alleviate the symptoms of acute altitude sickness. Sometimes one might have to descend to the altitude at which the symptoms first occurred to alleviate the symptoms.

HACE or HAPE

- This is extremely serious and treatment must be instituted immediately!
- If at all possible, **descend now.** The best treatment for HACE and HAPE is **descent, descent, descent!**
- Other treatment includes the administration of oxygen, pressure bags, and specialized medications. These may be necessary if descent is not possible.

Remember, the best medicine is prevention. Spending one or two nights at an intermediate altitude will help in acclimatization and preventing high altitude sickness. Do not ruin your vacation and incur the risk of serious illness or death by not taking time to acclimatize.
DESCEND! DESCEND! DESCEND!

For more information

1. *Altitude Illness: Prevention and Treatment.* Stephen Bezruchka M.D. (The Mountaineers, 2001).
2. http.//www.high-altitude-medicine.com.

CRUISE SHIPS

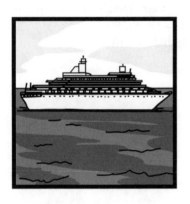

The growth of the cruise ship industry is a testament to the popularity of this type of vacation.

About six million people in the United States take a cruise vacation each year. About five percent of these people (about 300,000) seek medical attention while away on a cruise. Most of these medical problems are relatively minor in nature. Even though health care aboard cruise ships has recently improved, do not assume that every modern cruise ship has sophisticated medical care and medical facilities on board!

If you or your child has a significant medical problem, you should check prior to going on the cruise that the cruise ship has the medical capability to take care of these medical problems. Do not assume that you can be transported relatively easily to a sophisticated medical facility close by. Many of the locations that these cruise ships visit do **not** have sophisticated medical facilities.

Cruise ships are ideal locations for the spread of disease. They collect together people from many parts of the world in a confined environment. Some board with infectious diseases. Others are incubating them. The crew also often comes from widely diverse locations and frequently from developing countries where infectious diseases are common.

Illnesses most frequently encountered aboard cruise ships are:

- **Gastro intestinal illnesses,** notably travelers' diarrhea. Occasional outbreaks of hepatitis A have also been reported.

- **Respiratory tract infections,** mainly URIs (coughs and colds) but also influenza. Flu may occur even in the summer months as passengers from another hemisphere may import their flu with them!

- **Accidents,** principally minor falls. These are more common on the first day or two after boarding before you have had time to get your "sea legs."

- **Motion sickness.** See relevant section in this book.

As always, the best medicine is prevention.

- Before you leave, check whether the medical insurance you have back home will cover medical expenses incurred while aboard ship. They are not usually covered. Purchase traveler's **medical insurance with assistance.**

- Make sure your **immunizations** are up to date, especially for **hepatitis A.** Consider getting a **flu shot.**

- Pay attention to **safe food and water** precautions (see relevant section). When you disembark at the various ports on your voyage, eat wisely. Even on board ship, avoid high risk foods such as potato and egg salad, custards, and cream-filled pastries. Remember, much of the food served on the ship may have been taken on board at the last port of call. Wash hands before eating.

Despite all these warnings, most people do **not** get ill while on a cruise. They have a wonderful vacation with ample fresh air and sumptuous buffets. The cruise ship industry works hard to maintain good standards of hygiene. Medical care aboard cruise ships continues to improve.

Enjoy your trip!

TRAVELING WITH CHILDREN WITH CHRONIC ILLNESSES AND SPECIAL NEEDS

Traveling with children with chronic illnesses or special needs poses added challenges and additional preparation is necessary. If traveling to remote areas, reliable medical care may not be available and parents need to be certain that they are capable of handling their child's illness on their own. If not, select a different travel destination.

If you have a child with a chronic illness or medical problem, it is especially important to visit a travel clinic or travel physician before your travels.

It is essential that your child's immunizations are up-to-date and that you are adequately prepared to prevent such travel-related illnesses as travelers' diarrhea and malaria.

Many **airports** have upgraded their **security measures** because of the increase of the threat of terrorism. Consequently it is very important to check with the Federal Aviation Administration (FAA) and your airline if your child uses any **medical equipment** that you will need to take on board the aircraft. Do this **several days** before your departure date so that you have enough time to get any necessary letters, prescriptions etc. from your child's doctor to document the reasons your child needs to carry these items on board.

Asthma.

If your child has very unstable asthma and is prone to severe attacks of asthma, it is unwise to travel to countries with limited medical facilities. In fact, **it is not sensible to travel until asthma is under good control.**

While on vacation, your child's asthma may act up as he may be exposed to a variety of **asthma triggers**. These triggers include:

- Molds, which are very common in hot and humid environments and especially at seaside resorts. Many people have well controlled asthma until they open up their seaside cottage at the beginning of summer and are met with a barrage of mold spores!

- Upper respiratory infections picked up while traveling and being in confined spaces with many other people.

- Exposure to irritants such as cigarette smoke. This is common in buses, aircraft, trains, and public places in many countries.

- The excitement and the anxiety that often goes with travel.

- Forgetting to take medication because of the disruption in your child's usual routine.

Often a **combination of triggers** results in the worsening of your child's asthma.

Discuss with your child's doctor whether your child's asthma medication needs to be increased prior to and while away on travel. This applies particularly to the **controller** (preventer) medications such as inhaled corticosteroids. Make sure you take along sufficient medication, especially sufficient **"rescue"** medication such as albuterol or other short-acting bronchodilators and a course of **oral steroids**. All of this should be discussed with your doctor prior to travel. You should have with you a **written asthma action plan** outlining the steps to be taken in the event that your child has an asthma attack or your child's asthma symptoms increase.

It is always better to err on the side of being overcautious and to overtreat rather than undertreat asthma, especially while away on vacation or in unfamiliar surroundings.

Early signs that asthma may be getting out of control are a **cough** late at night (10 PM to 2 AM) and a cough with exercise. If your child needs to use his "rescue" inhaler more often than usual, this suggests that the asthma is worsening. A person with well controlled asthma should not need to use their "rescue" inhaler more than twice a week! On the other hand, wheezing may come on suddenly if your child is exposed to inhaled allergens such as peanut dust on board the airplane.

Keep your child's asthma medication, especially the "rescue" medication with you at all times. Older children should carry their medication with them.

Younger children who usually receive their medication by nebulizers requiring a source of electricity, may do very well on meter-dose inhalers (MDIs) administered with the aid of a spacer or holding chamber. However, if any changes are to be made, these changes should be made some time before your departure and your physician should check on your child's technique when using MDIs and spacers.

Diabetes.

Travel, even travel to far off and lesser developed lands, is not contraindicated if your child has diabetes, as long as your child's diabetes is stable. You should also have a good understanding of the illness, diabetic medication, and how to recognize and treat the complications of diabetes, including hypoglycemia and hyperglycemia. Even if you have a good understanding of your child's diabetes, it is preferable to select countries that have good medical care.

It is not wise to travel with a newly diagnosed diabetic as the insulin requirements vary greatly and you are unlikely to be familiar enough with the necessary adjustments in insulin dosage. There are many facets to the care of a diabetic and it takes time to get a good understanding of the disease.

Your child's diabetes will probably be more difficult to control while traveling due to a combination of factors:

- Irregular meal times.
- Different foods, not all of which may be to your child's liking and so may not be eaten!
- Motion sickness.
- Excitement.
- Variable exercise levels. It is impossible to get sufficient exercise on a long flight. On the other hand, once you are sight-seeing or hiking, your child may be exercising far more than usual.
- Change in time zones and sleep patterns.
- Illnesses such as upper respiratory infections, travelers' diarrhea, etc.

Things to do _before_ departure

1. **Visit** your **child's diabetes** physician or **diabetic educator** and discuss your proposed travels with him or her.

    - Request a letter stating that she has diabetes and will need to carry syringes, needles, and medications with her. This letter must be written on **office letterhead.**

    - Get **prescriptions** for all your child's medicines, syringes, etc. In order to board with syringes and other insulin delivery devices, you must produce an insulin vial with a professional, pharmaceutical, pre-printed label that clearly identifies the medication. If the prescription is on the outside of the box that the insulin comes in, you should carry that as well.

- Get a **contact phone number** that you can use for advice after hours and over weekends (most diabetics already have this). Remember, you may be calling from a different time zone.

- Ask for guidelines on adjusting insulin doses if you plan on crossing many time zones (more than four times zones).

- If your child's usual insulin regimen does not include short acting insulin such as *humalog,* ask for a prescription for this and guidance on how to use it. *This insulin has a rapid onset and short duration of action. It is ideal when your child may need extra doses of insulin when crossing time zones or when your schedule, meal times and exercise are unpredictable and erratic.*

- Insulin pen injectors have insulin containing cartridges which make the administration of insulin far more convenient while traveling.

Note: Any changes in your child's insulin regimen should be made weeks before travel and not just before you depart.

2. **Contact the FAA and the American Diabetes Association** (http://www.diabetes.org.) to find out the latest recommendations regarding guidelines and restrictions concerning the carriage of medical equipment on board the aircraft. (You may take lancets on board if they are capped and they are carried with a glucose meter with the manufacturer's name embossed on the meter).

3. Make sure you have an **adequate supply** of insulin, insulin syringes, glucagon, glucose test strips, and an extra battery for the blood glucose meter (glucometer) or a spare meter. Include ketone urine test strips to detect and monitor ketones in the urine. **It is a good**

idea to take extra quantities of insulin and other supplies in case there are unscheduled delays or other mishaps. Most authorities recommend that you take at least double the supplies you think you will need. You may not be able to purchase the identical insulin in other countries.

4. If your child uses an **insulin pump** and you are traveling outside the United States, either take along a supply of insulin and syringes, or contact your pump company and request a **back-up loaner** in case the pump fails. Also, take along your pump manual and log book with basal rates. Insulin pumps are **not** harmed by metal detectors and will not trigger the airport metal detectors.

5. If you intend to travel to extreme climates, purchase an appropriate **container** in which **to carry your child's insulin** (Contact Medicool Insulin Protector at (800) 433-2469). Although insulin does not have to be refrigerated it is not a good idea to expose it to extremes of temperature. It may not do well in the aircraft hold where it may freeze, or in the desert sun! Consider purchasing an appropriate carrying case to carry all your child's diabetic medication and equipment. **Keep this with you while traveling.**

6. Purchase a **supply of snacks** to treat low blood sugars or to take the place of meals that do not meet your child's fancy.

7. If your child is prone to **motion sickness,** purchase medication to prevent this. (See chapter on motion sickness.)

8. It is **especially important to visit a travel clinic or travel physician** if you intend to travel to countries where contracting illnesses such as travelers' diarrhea or malaria are likely.

- Get appropriate advice on the prevention and treatment of malaria and travelers' diarrhea, etc.
- Get appropriate immunizations, including a flu shot and the pneumococcal vaccine.
- Get further advice about medical facilities and diseases relevant to the countries you intend to visit.

9. Make sure you have extra **travel insurance.** If you are traveling to remote or lesser developed countries, consider purchasing **evacuation insurance** as well.

10. Make sure you know how to locate reliable health care while away (see appropriate section in the book). The American Diabetes Association and the International Diabetes Federation (http://www.idf.org) may also be able to provide you with additional information and medical contacts while away. Contact these organizations prior to departure and keep the phone numbers and addresses in a safe place with your other documents. If you have a Medtronic MiniMed insulin pump, contact Medtronic to get the direct phone numbers to Medtronic MiniMed because the 800 number will not work outside the United States. The general phone number is (818) 362-5958. The 24-hour helpline is (818) 576-5555. Medtronic MiniMed has offices worldwide and can assist you in locating an endocrinologist internationally.

11. You may also want to phone the airline and order your child diabetic meals for the flight.

While traveling

- Ensure your child wears her diabetic identification bracelet (medic alert bracelet) at all times.

- **Keep all you child's diabetic medication and equipment with you in your carry-on luggage.**

- **Make sure you always have a supply of snacks with you.** This is especially important while traveling, as you may not know when you child's next meal will be.

- Carry with you, on your person, a letter from your child's doctor stating that she has diabetes and will need to carry her medication, syringes, and needles with her at all times. **Have this letter easily accessible** at check-in and available for airport security.

- Try to regulate your child's meals as much as possible. If your child is taking her insulin in relation to meals, do not give insulin unless you are sure that her next meal is right in front of her.

- While flying, keep your watch set to the local time of your departure point while flying. This will help you keep track of the time in relation to your child's insulin schedule.

- If your child is prone to motion sickness, try to prevent this (see appropriate section in the book). If she has trouble keeping her meals down, it is far better to avoid large doses of long acting insulin. Rather use small frequent doses of short- acting insulin such as *humalog*.

  — You may need to adjust your child's insulin dosage if you will be crossing many (greater than four) time zones. When traveling west, the day will be longer and your child may need an extra dose of insulin. When traveling east, the opposite happens—the day will be shorter. Your child may therefore need less insulin, especially long-acting insulin. You should have discussed all this with your child's diabetic physician prior to travel.

178 ◆ PEDIATRIC HEALTH PROBLEMS

— **The secret to diabetic control while traveling is to check your child's blood glucose level more frequently.** This cannot be emphasized enough.

— You should not aim to keep as tight control as you do at home, but aim to avoid the extremes—too high blood glucose or even more importantly, too low blood glucose. You may decide to let your child's blood glucose run a little higher than usual to avoid hypoglycemia.

Other points to note while traveling

• Be on the lookout for scratches and insect bites which, in a diabetic child tend to become infected more easily. Clean scratches, abrasions, and bites well and apply an anti-itch ointment and possibly a topical antibiotic as well. Keep your child's nails short to prevent further skin damage from scratching.

• Good **foot care** is essential. If your child is doing a lot of walking or hiking keep an eye on your child's feet to make sure that blisters are avoided. This is not the time to try out new boots! Treat any foot problems early.

• Be especially vigilant regarding **safe food and water precautions.** It is important to prevent travelers' diarrhea in diabetics, as diarrhea and vomiting will make your child's diabetes more difficult to control.

• Make sure your child drinks plenty of fluids and keeps well hydrated. Keep an eye on her urine output (both color and amount). This is especially important in hot climates and while hiking or climbing.

- Glucose meters may not give reliable readings at high altitudes.

In summary, it is safe for most diabetic children to travel, provided the diabetes is under good control and provided they are supervised well during their travels. Do not aim for extremely tight control but **do check your child's blood glucose levels more frequently** and anticipate events that are likely to put your child's diabetes out of control, such as erratic meals times, motion sickness, travelers' diarrhea, etc.

Children with chronic lung disease and cardiac disease.

If your child has serious cardiac disease or chronic lung disease, discuss the suitability of air travel with your child's physician. Extra oxygen may be required during the flight. Commercial airlines will not allow private oxygen tanks aboard the aircraft but will supply oxygen if contacted in advance.

If you plan to travel to high altitude locations, have your child checked beforehand by a pulmonologist (lung specialist) and a cardiologist (heart specialist) and discuss with them the advisability of traveling to such a location. A child with chronic lung disease (other than asthma) and some cardiac diseases are especially prone to high altitude sickness.

Children with recurrent chronic ear problems.

See relevant section on ears and flying.

Children in wheelchairs

Contact the airlines to make appropriate wheelchair and transport arrangements. Some countries are not suitable for handicapped people and you should research this beforehand. Most barriers are not insurmountable but the stresses and hassles of travel will be increased.

Epilepsy.

Make sure your child's epilepsy is well controlled prior to travel. If indicated, have anticonvulsant blood levels checked. Take an adequate supply of medication, including medication to treat seizures acutely (such as **rectal *Diazepam***). Be sure you know how to use this medication. Discuss this with your child's physician beforehand and write down the directions and dosages.

Children with colostomy bags and intestinal disorders

Take along an adequate supply of colostomy supplies as they may not be obtainable in other countries or may not be the right size. Be sure to apply a larger than usual bag when flying as the air inside the bag will tend to expand with air travel. Using a larger bag may prevent leakage.

If your child has diarrhea and needs to go to the bathroom frequently, as many people with ulcerative colitis do, **reserve an aisle seat.** This will definitely make the flight less stressful for everyone!

Children with intestinal disorders such as Crohn's disease, ulcerative colitis, celiac disease, short gut, etc., are more prone to travelers' diarrhea. If they get travelers' diarrhea it is more likely to be severe and possibly lead to dehydration. It is especially important for these children to be **vigilant regarding safe food and water precautions** to avoid travelers' diarrhea. It may be wise for these children to be on **prophylactic antibiotics** for travelers' diarrhea or possibly to take *Pepto-Bismol* on a regular basis. If they are not already on an antibiotic, it is a good idea for these children to have access to an appropriate antibiotic in the event that they do develop travelers' diarrhea. Discuss this with your child's physician prior to departure and take along the necessary medication.

If your child is taking medication to suppress gastric acid production or is on medication to treat gastroesophageal reflux (regurgitation of stomach contents up the esophagus), he may be more prone to travelers' diarrhea. Prophylactic antibiotics or prophylactic *Pepto-Bismol* may be indicated.

BRINGING YOUR INTERNATIONALLY ADOPTED CHILD HOME

OVERVIEW

What you need to do before you collect your child.

- Visit *your* physician or a travel clinic
- Visit your *child's* future physician. Discuss—
  - — Medications and supplies you should take with you.
  - — What to do if your child is ill when you collect her.
- Contact a family who has adopted a child from the same country.
- Get non-medical supplies you may need for your newly adopted child.
- Get supplies for the parents and traveling siblings.

Common medical issues encountered in foreign adoptees.

Things to be aware of while you are in your adopted child's country.

Many U.S. citizens adopt children from outside the United States, commonly from China, Russia, and Romania, but also from many other countries. Finally, after months or years of waiting, it is time for you to collect your child and bring him or her home! This is obviously a very exciting time for you and your family. Remember, you may be traveling to a lesser-developed country and you should plan appropriately. You do not want to spoil this special time by becoming ill. Your adoption agency will have provided you with helpful information about the country you will be visiting and will possibly have given you recommendations for preventing travel-related illness.

You have a number of things to do before you collect your child.

1. Visit *your* physician or a travel clinic.

Especially if you are traveling to a lesser-developed country, it is **essential** that you get advice to guide you, particularly in regard to the prevention of travel-related illness. Make sure your immunizations are up-to-date, especially against **hepatitis A and B** and know how to prevent and treat travelers' diarrhea. **This visit should take place three to six months prior to your departure date to allow sufficient time for your immunizations.** However, if you have left it to the last moment, still make this appointment as you may be able to prevent some very unpleasant illnesses!

If you are traveling to an area where malaria is prevalent, you will need to take precautions to prevent mosquito bites and you may also need to take prophylactic anti-malarial medication.

Sometimes adopting parents take their own parents with them to share this exciting time or perhaps to help take care of siblings. If an elderly person accompanies you, it is especially important that he or she has travel insurance and has visited a travel clinic for advice and assessment. Elderly people should also get the **pneumovax immunization** which gives protection against a very severe type of pneumonia. It is also a good idea for the elderly to get a **flu shot.** It is actually a good idea for everyone to get a flu shot!

Do <u>not</u> bypass this visit!

2. **Visit your *child's* future physician.**

You may have already met with your child's future physician to review the adoption records, your child's growth and development charts, etc. Even if you have already met, another visit to discuss the following issues is a good idea.

➤ **A) A list of medications and supplies to take with you.**

- Analgesics and antipyretics such as acetaminophen (*Tylenol*) and ibuprofen (children's *Motrin* and children's *Advil*). (See section 1: A Pediatric Medical Kit, for dosages.)

- Diaper rash ointments and creams such as *A & D, Desitin,* or *Triple Paste*.

- Antifungal creams or ointments such as *Nystatin* (prescription) or clotrimazole (*Lotrimin*).

- Antibacterial ointment such as *triple antibiotic, Neosporin, Bacitracin,* or *Bactroban* (prescription).

- Hydrocortisone cream, either ½% or 1% to treat itchy rashes, insect bites, or contact dermatitis.

- *Elimite* cream to treat scabies (prescription).

- *Nix cream rinse* and a nit comb to treat head lice.

- Saline nose drops with a bulb syringe.

- Allergy medication such as *Benadryl* to treat itching, allergic reactions, and colds (for *Benadryl* dosage, see section 1: A Pediatric Medical Kit).

- Laxatives such as glycerine suppositories or *Babylax.*
- Rehydration salts such as *Kaolectrolyte, Pedialyte,* or *Ceralyte.* These need to be mixed with clean, drinkable water. Remember, if there is any doubt about the safety of the water, it should be boiled or treated chemically before use (see chapter on preparation of safe water).
- A thermometer.
- Vaseline to lubricate the thermometer (if used rectally) or to treat dry, chapped skin and lips.
- A course of antibiotics (prescription).
- Antibiotic ear drops (prescription).
- Antibiotic eye drops (prescription).

The last three suggestions are optional extras. Some physicians recommend these and others do not. Discuss these with your child's physician before you depart and get clear guidelines as to when the antibiotics should be used. Know the correct dose for your child.

NOTE: Most parents have medical and developmental questions about their future child. Some parents undertake an initial **first look visit** to assess their prospective child. If you are one of these parents, it is a good idea to meet with a pediatrician beforehand. A pediatrician can give you guidelines on what to look for, how to assess development, how to measure a child's head size (head circumference), and how to plot a child's measurements on a percentile chart. If you are planning such a visit, take the following with you:

— Percentile charts.

— A Denver developmental chart.

— A tape measure to measure head circumference.

— A camcorder to video your child.

None of this will qualify you to assess a child accurately, but armed with this information plus birth and developmental history, a pediatrician that specializes in adoption can help you assess a child. Remember, there are **no** guarantees!

There are many clinics and services that specialize in foreign adoptions. One such service can be accessed at http://www.adoptionsinternational.com.

➢ **B)** **What to do if your child is ill when you collect her.**

Usually the orphanage will be able to suggest a local physician to take care of the problem. Failing this, the U.S. Embassy may be able to recommend a physician. Alternatively, your child's future physician may be prepared to accept a long-distance call from you to discuss the problem and advise you. Some agencies specializing in foreign adoption may be able to give you the phone numbers of local physicians in specific locations who are very qualified to help you take care of your child's problems. If you are working through such an agency, get the names and phone numbers **before** you leave home.

As part of the exit procedure your child will require a physical examination to acquire a U.S. visa. This examination is usually fairly cursory and certainly does not take the place of a full medical evaluation when you get home.

3. Contact a family who has adopted a child from the same country.

It is a good idea to contact a family who has already adopted a child and discuss their experience. You could ask them what they would do differently if they were to do it again.

There are a number of websites where you can chat with other families who have already adopted children internationally. Such a website is http://www.rainbowkids.com.

4. Get non-medical supplies you may need for your newly adopted child.

- Formula: Depending upon the country you are visiting, it may be a good idea to take along three or four cans of infant formula. This could be a regular milk-based formula or a soy-based formula. Although many Asian individuals are lactose intolerant, this usually only develops later in life, and consequently lactose intolerance is not usually a problem. Do not make too many changes to your child's routine when you first receive her. Keep her on the formula or milk she is used to. This applies to the other elements of her diet as well. You will have ample time when you get back to transition her to a different type of formula, or, if she is older than one year of age, to whole milk.

- Other important items to take along are disposable diapers, wet wipes, toilet paper, and clothing. The orphanage will gratefully accept any items not used! The orphanage will also happily accept any medications that you do not need.

- Stickers, books, and toys. *One adopting parent told me of an intriguing way in which she got her new child to make eye contact. She placed a sticker on her nose and one her child's nose and they had great fun looking at each other and laughing.*

5. **Get supplies for the parents and traveling siblings.** These are detailed elsewhere in the book, and include basic analgesics, routine medications that you take, and medications to prevent and treat travelers' diarrhea. If you are traveling to a malarial area, anti-malarial precautions will need to be followed. If you are prone to constipation, include a suitable laxative in your medical kit.

   If you are traveling to an area where SARS or some other similar contagious disease is known to occur, consider purchasing N-95 masks.

   If you arrive jet-lagged and are unable to sleep, sleeping tablets may help you get a few good nights sleep before you collect your child. *Ambien* (zoldipem) is a suitable sleeping tablet. This is a prescription medication so discuss this with your own doctor.

Common medical issues encountered in foreign adoptees.

Skin

- **Mongolian spots**
  These are blue-green or slate grey marks in the skin, particularly over the lower back. They are common in more deeply pigmented races, especially blacks and Asians. These marks may be mistaken for bruises. They often fade in later childhood.

- **Dry skin/eczema**

  Many adoptees have dry skin and sometimes patches of eczema (atopic dermatitis). These patches are usually worse on the cheeks but may occur anywhere. Sometimes the patches of eczema have a circular shape and may be mistaken for ringworm. Some children may have cracked and bleeding skin behind the ears.

  If your child scratches enough, the skin may be scratched open and start bleeding. Secondary infection may occur. When this happens, the infected areas are called impetigo. (See section on atopic dermatitis/eczema.)

- **Impetigo**

  Impetigo, an infection of the skin due to bacteria (streptococci or staphylococci), is also relatively common and often follows scratching of bug bites and eczema. (See section on impetigo.)

- **Bug bites**

  Bug bites are particularly common in children living in hot and humid countries. (See section on bug bites.)

- **Scabies**

  Scabies is seen quite frequently in children in developing countries, including adoptees. It is also not rare in children and adults in the United States. If your child is scratching continuously and has red bumps over parts of her body, then she may have scabies. This is particularly likely if others in the orphanage have similar symptoms. These red bumps occur particularly on the hands and feet, between the fingers and toes, but also on the outer aspect of the hands and feet and around the wrists and ankles.

  If you suspect scabies, apply the *Elimite* cream from head to toe, and leave on for eight to twelve hours. Your child should then be bathed and the *Elimite* washed off.

Dress your child in clean clothing Your child is likely to continue scratching for some time afterwards. *Benadryl* may help reduce the itch. Further treatment or a second *Elimite* treatment may be applied once you return home.

Scabies is very contagious so if you do not treat your child soon, you will develop scabies! You will know this because you will be itching! Scabies in adults is often most severe where clothing comes into contact with the skin, especially where bra straps or the elastic of underpants comes into contact with the skin.

• **Lice (nits)**
Nits in the hair are not unusual in the U.S.A. They are more common in lesser developed countries and especially in children from orphanages or institutions.

The most common symptom of lice is itchiness of the scalp. You may see the adult lice moving in your child's hair, but you are more likely to see the eggs (the nits) attached to strands of hair. They are most commonly seen behind the ears and at the nape of the neck close to the scalp. They may be mistaken for dandruff but dandruff is easily brushed off or combed out.

A good medication for treating lice is *Nix crème rinse*. This is applied as follows: Wash the hair with a regular shampoo. Towel off excess water so that the hair is damp but not wet and then apply enough *Nix* to soak the hair and scalp. Pay particular attention to the area behind the ears and the nape of the neck. Wash off the *Nix* after ten minutes. Rinse the hair well with water.

• **Ringworm**
Circular skin lesions with a dry, scaly edge may be due to ringworm. Use an antifungal cream such as *Lotrimin* to treat this. They may take weeks to disappear. As mentioned above, eczema is often misdiagnosed as ringworm.

Fever

Remember, most fevers are due to mild viral infections which are usually not serious. (See section on fever.)

Ear infections and upper respiratory tract infections (URIs)

Children everywhere have frequent colds and "runny noses" and international adoptees are no exception! Do not be alarmed if your child has yellow or green mucus streaming from her nose. (See section on colds/URIs.)

Some children may have pus draining out of one or both ears. This indicates they have an ear infection and the ear drum has ruptured. Children in lesser developed countries commonly have this problem which is known medically as "chronic suppurative otitis media." This does not usually cause pain or discomfort and does not have to be treated immediately. Treatment usually includes drying up the pus with many Q-tips and instilling antibiotic ear drops (such as *Floxin* or *Ciprodex*), two to three times a day for many days. Sometimes an oral antibiotic is also used. If the draining ear is a recent event, it suggests the ear infection has just occurred and an antibiotic by mouth is the appropriate treatment. (See section on ear infections.)

Coughs

Coughs commonly accompany a cold. There are many other causes for a cough, most of which are not serious. (See section on coughs.)

Eye problems

Your child may have "pink eye" or a pussy eye when you fetch her. This is known as conjunctivitis. (See section on "pink eye"/conjunctivitis.)

Gastro-intestinal problems

- **Vomiting.**
  The occasional vomit or "spit-up" is normal in childhood. If vomiting is more severe it may require treatment (See section on vomiting.)

- **Constipation**
  Constipation is common in children and adults, especially when traveling. (See section on constipation.)

- **Loose Stools and Diarrhea**
  These are also not unusual. Both constipation and diarrhea may be exacerbated by changes in diet and emotional stress. (See sections on diarrhea and dehydration and travelers' diarrhea.)

Most of the illnesses you encounter will be minor. Do not panic. There is usually no hurry to treat them. If you are concerned, call you child's physician at home and ask for advice. Occasionally your child will have a serious problem that will need to be treated urgently. As a physician who treats many international adoptees, I am constantly heartened by the health and good nutrition of most of the children who enter the United States.

Things to be aware of while you are in your adopted child's country and while waiting to return to the United States.

- This is a stressful time but also a very special time. Do not try to do too much. Don't feel you have to sightsee. Get as much sleep as possible and try to keep a sense of humor and enjoy this happy time.

- Eat sensibly. Remember your travelers' diarrhea precautions. Watch out for constipation.

- You and your new child may be spending many hours in a hotel room. There may be safety concerns here—loose and unprotected electrical wires, windows that open easily to the road below, bathroom hazards such as very hot water. Don't forget about choking and poisoning. Your child's inquisitive fingers may reach medicines not intended for her.

Collecting an international adoptee is extremely exciting but also exhausting and stressful. Making the appropriate preparations, being well rested prior to travel, and not being rushed will help make the entire visit more enjoyable.

Once you have returned home, and you and your new child have had time to settle and adapt to the new time zone, you should make an appointment for your child to have a full physical examination. Later your child will need some screening blood tests, possibly a chest x-ray, and some stool tests. Some of the blood tests may need to be repeated six months later. Immunizations will also need to be administered at some stage.

Congratulations!

SARS: SEVERE ACUTE RESPIRATORY SYNDROME

Severe acute respiratory syndrome (SARS) is an illness which was first described in the winter of 2003. It began in Vietnam and China but spread fairly rapidly to other countries around the world, including the United States and Canada.

SARS is a **viral disease** which probably originated in animals but the virus is able to thrive in humans as well. During the 2003 outbreak over 8,000 people worldwide developed SARS and there were over eight hundred deaths due to the disease. Most of the people infected were adults but a few children also became ill with the disease. **Health care workers** appeared to be particularly vulnerable. By August 2003, the disease appeared to be contained with no new cases being diagnosed. Only time will tell whether SARS will reemerge every winter.

How do you get SARS?

SARS is acquired by **close contact** with someone who already has the disease or by touching objects contaminated with the virus. "Close contact" means living or taking care of someone with SARS. It would also include sharing eating and drinking utensils, touching the individual (shaking hands, kissing or hugging) and talking to someone within three feet.

How long is the incubation period?

The incubation period may be as short as five days or as long as fifteen days.

What are the symptoms of SARS?

The early symptoms of SARS are similar to many other infectious illnesses and include fever, headache, muscle aches and often diarrhea. Later on (after two to seven days), the person may develop a cough and shortness of breath. If an x-ray is taken at this stage it will show pneumonia. Some people may be only mildly ill while others will be critically ill and require hospitalization, extra oxygen, intravenous fluids, and highly skilled medical and nursing care. Antibiotics will **not** kill the SARS virus (antibiotics do not kill viruses), but may be indicated for other reasons.

How is the diagnosis of SARS made?

This is **not** an easy diagnosis to make as it is very similar to many other types of pneumonia. It is suspected if the ill person has recently had contact with a known case or has recently traveled to an area where SARS is prevalent. Laboratories around the world are working on more specific and accurate tests for SARS but most of these are either experimental or available only at a few highly specialized research laboratories.

How can I avoid contracting SARS?

Be sensible! Avoid unnecessary travel to areas that are experiencing SARS outbreaks. The CDC issues *travel advisories and alerts*. A **travel advisory** recommends that nonessential travel be deferred. A **travel alert** does not advise against travel, but informs travelers of a health concern and provides advice about specific precautions. The CDC website for SARS is http://www.cdc.gov/.

What did we learn from the SARS outbreak?

- **We learned how quickly infectious illnesses can spread around the world.** With the advent of jet travel, a disease may be in China one day and the United States the next! There is no longer just "the slow boat to China"! We are all brothers and sisters on a very small planet and need to respect and take care of each other.

- **We learned if we work together we can solve complex medical questions much faster and stop the spread of disease.** In the case of SARS, the World Health Organization (WHO) and laboratories around the world worked together to detect the SARS virus and contain the disease. **Cooperation instead of competition between nations makes the world a better and safer place!**

SARS may or may not have gone, but other new infectious diseases will surely arise from time to time. Below are some sensible general measures to decrease your chances of getting contagious diseases.

General measures to avoid contracting infectious diseases

- **Avoid traveling to areas experiencing outbreaks of disease.** This is not always possible as you may already be in an area when a disease outbreak occurs. Alternatively, you may have to travel to areas experiencing epidemics for personal or other reasons. This happened during the SARS outbreak when many westerners chose to travel to areas of China where SARS was prevalent to collect their newly adopted children. Consult the CDC or your travel clinic to learn about high-risk areas.

- If traveling to areas where a communicable disease has broken out, **avoid contact with large numbers of people.**
- **Wash your hands frequently.** Doorknobs, handrails and elevator buttons may all be contaminated. You may not always have access to running water so have easily accessible a bottle of **bactericidal hand sanitizer lotion** or **alcohol-based wet wipes.** Use these regularly.
- Try to limit close contact with strangers. Avoid kissing, hugging, and even shaking hands.
- **Do not share eating and drinking utensils.**
- **What about masks?** If you have close contact with an infected person, masks may be helpful. So may eye glasses or goggles. One of the ways these help is to help you cut down the number of times you rub your eyes or touch your nose. Wearing a mask often suggests to other people that you have some terrible and contagious disease. Masks may help by discouraging other people from coming too close to you! An N-95 mask is one of the more effective types of mask.
- **What about surgical gloves?** These may help too but often give a false sense of security. Even if you are wearing gloves, if you touch infected material and then rub your eyes or scratch your nose, you stand a good chance of transferring the infected material to yourself.
- **If you get sick** while traveling or soon after returning home **seek expert medical attention.** When you make your appointment, tell your health care provider

that you have recently been in an area that has an outbreak of an infectious disease. Health care workers can then take the necessary precautions to avoid contracting the disease and spreading it to other patients.

- **Wash your hands! Wash your hands! Wash your hands!**

3

Common Childhood Illnesses and Their Symptoms

THE NEWBORN INFANT AND INFANTS IN THE FIRST TWO TO THREE MONTHS OF LIFE

One of the most exciting things that can happen to one is to bring home a newborn baby! Babies do not come with instruction manuals, and one's excitement is often mixed with a certain amount of anxiety. Discussed below are some of the unusual but normal things babies do.

Skin.

Skin color
Newborn infants and infants in the first few months of life often have very blue, even purple, hands and feet. Sometimes the upper lip has a bluish tinge. This is due to poor circulation and is normal. However, your infant's tongue should be nice and pink.

The skin in the first week or ten days of life frequently is **yellowish** in color. The whites of the eyes may also be yellow. This is known as **jaundice** and is due to a substance called bilirubin that is found in excess in many newborn babies. Although this is not usually a problem, it is important to have an infant checked in the first week of life to make sure that the level of bilirubin in the body is not too high—a very high level of bilirubin can cause brain damage.

Rashes

Although babies are usually born with a lovely soft skin, after a few days it often becomes dry and cracked and may even bleed in certain areas (particularly around the ankles). No treatment is usually necessary, but you can decrease the dryness by bathing your infant less frequently or by applying a hypoallergenic moisturizer to the skin. It is normal for the skin to peel.

Babies have very sensitive skin and develop a variety of rashes, which tend to come and go. They often have reddish bumps with a yellowish-white center scattered over the body. (The medical term for this rash is *erythema toxicum.*) These spots last for a week or two and are usually of no consequence apart from the fact that they may be mistaken for infected pustules.

Neonatal acne

Small pimples on the face that resemble acne are known as neonatal or newborn acne. **Neonatal acne** usually develops around the third or fourth week of life, is common, requires no treatment and may last for many months. White spots on the nose are called **milia** and are also normal.

"Stork bites"

Many infants are born with reddish or pinkish marks or blotches on the upper eyelids, base of the nose and nape of the neck. These are known as salmon patches or "stork bites" and usually fade with time (months to years).

Diaper rashes

Diaper rashes are common, and are best prevented by keeping the genital area clean and dry. If your infant develops a rash in the diaper area, apply a barrier ointment, such as *Desitin, A & D,* or *Triple Paste.* If this does not clear the rash in two to three days, then try an antifungal ointment such as *Nystatin* or *Lotrimin.*

Good hygiene is the most important way to prevent and treat diaper rash, so change your child's diaper as soon as he or she is wet or dirty. You may need to wash your baby with warm water and a mild soap. Do not use plastic pants because they tend to retain moisture and make diaper rashes worse. Most diaper rashes respond well to air. (See section on diaper rashes.)

When to Contact a Physician

Occasionally, a rash in an infant may be a sign of a more serious underlying disease.

- Large blisters may be a sign of a serious underlying illness.
- If your infant has a non-blanching rash (a rash that does not fade when you press on it) and is acting ill (lethargic, decreased drinking, fever, etc.), it is important that you consult with a physician immediately.
- Redness around the umbilicus that is spreading outward over the belly area indicates an urgent need to visit a physician.

Breathing.

Newborn babies often **sneeze,** and this does not mean they are getting a cold or have allergies. They will often sound very "snuffly" from breathing through narrow nasal passages that contain mucus. If this interferes with feeding, it may be helpful to instill salt-water (saline) nose drops and to suction the mucus with a bulb syringe. Do one nostril at a time. Your infant will object to this procedure, but it is effective. If the mucus contains a small amount of blood, don't be concerned. These nose drops may be purchased over the counter (*Nasal, Little Noses, Ocean, Altamist*) or made up at home (dissolve 1/2 level tsp. of table salt in 8 oz. water).

Babies often make a lot of noise when they breathe. You will find this out if your baby sleeps in the same room as you! They also do not breathe nice and evenly. They often have periods of very rapid breathing and then hold their breath for ten to fifteen seconds. This can be very disconcerting if your infant is sleeping right next to you. You may find yourself jumping out of bed to check if your child is still breathing!

How fast do babies breathe? In the first few months of life, babies take forty or more breaths a minute. At times, particularly after crying or feeding they may breathe seventy or eighty or more times a minute! However, once they have settled, the respiratory rate should be around forty times a minute or less.

Eyes.

As mentioned above, the whites of a newborn's eyes often are yellow due to jaundice. This may last for one to three weeks, or even longer but is no cause for concern if your baby's bilirubin level is not too high.

Some babies have red streaks in the whites of one or both eyes. These are hemorrhages, occur during the birthing process and fade over the ensuing two to three weeks.

"Sticky" or pussy eyes: This may be due to an eye infection (**conjunctivitis**) or to **blocked tear ducts**. The latter often leads to excessive watering of the eyes. If your baby's eyelids are red and swollen or are stuck together, he should be seen by a doctor. If there is just a small amount of discharge or they are just tearing excessively, discuss this with your child's doctor at his next check-up.

Your baby's "soft spot."

Your baby will have a large "soft spot" (the anterior fontanelle) at the top of the head toward the front. This spot will get smaller over time and is usually closed by age eighteen months. The soft spot is usually slightly depressed but sometimes it may appear fuller and tenser (for example, when a baby is lying down and crying or straining).

When to Contact a Physician

- A soft spot that is very sunken may be a sign of dehydration. If your infant is dehydrated there will be other signs of dehydration. (See section on dehydration).
- A tense, bulging fontanelle may be a sign of meningitis. In this case, your baby will also have a fever and be very irritable or very lethargic: seek immediate medical help!

Mouth and tongue.

A baby's tongue will often have a white coating on it, which can be wiped off easily. Usually the coating is just milk curds and typically occurs after feeding.

When to Contact a Physician

If the white coating extends to the inside of the cheeks, the gums, and the inside of the lips, and continues for some hours after a feed, your baby probably has thrush. Occasionally thrush can interfere with feeding and cause fussiness. Thrush is a fungal infection that often needs treatment with an oral antifungal medicine. Discuss this with your child's physician. Thrush is not a medical emergency and may get better on its own.

Spitting up/vomiting.

It is quite common for infants in the first few weeks of life to "spit-up." Sometimes when babies spit up the milk comes out through the nostrils! Do not be alarmed if this happens.

Many babies continue to spit-up throughout the first year of life. **As long as a baby is otherwise well, gaining weight, and happy, this is no cause for concern.** The medical terminology for this is gastro-esophageal reflux. Reflux tends to increase in severity and peaks at four months of age. It has usually resolved by one year of age. As a parent, while you have a baby around, there is not much point in wearing expensive silk shirts or blouses!

Some infants will have the occasional **projectile vomit** in which the vomit shoots out a few feet or more!

When to Contact a Physician

- If your infant has repeated projectile vomits that seem to get more severe and occur with increasing frequency, contact your child's physician.
- Any infant who "spits-ups" or vomits and does not gain weight adequately should be seen by a physician. So should an infant that is always unhappy and fussy.
- If your newborn infant vomits green-colored liquid (bile), then medical attention should be sought immediately.

The umbilicus (the "belly button" cord).

It is important to keep the cord (umbilicus) clean and dry. Many physicians recommend cleaning the cord three or four times a day with rubbing alcohol. This is probably not necessary; allowing the cord to dry naturally is just as effective.

The cord falls off within the first two to three weeks of life, but occasionally stays on for up to two months. When the cord falls off, you may see a drop or two of blood around the umbilicus, which is not a cause for alarm.

As mentioned earlier, redness of the skin at the base of the cord is **not** normal and may indicate a serious infection. Sometimes the cord develops an unpleasant odor but apart from the odor this is not usually a problem

Genitalia.

Boys

No special care is needed for the uncircumcised male penis. It is especially important **not** to retract the foreskin forcibly.

Circumcised males often develop redness, swelling, a yellowish crust, and oozing at the circumcision site in the first week or ten days after circumcision. The tip of the penis may look like it is infected, but this is normal at this stage. By ten to fourteen days the penis should be completely healed.

Girls

Girls may have a whitish vaginal discharge in the first week of life, and sometimes this is blood-tinged. This is no cause for alarm and will settle by ten days of age. You should clean the genital area with a cotton ball and warm water. When cleaning the genital area, always wipe from front to back.

Weight loss and weight gain.

All babies lose weight in the first few days of life. This is especially true of breast-fed babies because it may take up to a week for the mother's milk to come in fully. By seven to ten days of age, a baby should be back to his or her birth weight. After that your baby should gain five to seven ounces every week for the next two to three months. Most infants double their birth weight by four to five months and triple it by their first birthday.

Bowel movements.

Your infant's initial bowel movements may be almost black in color. These first stools are known as **meconium.**

The **stool color** may vary from bright yellow to bright green to brown or be various shades in between. Sometimes the stools have a seedy texture.

Breast-fed babies

Breast-fed babies may have seven to ten loose to watery stools a day. A stool is often passed each time the infant feeds. As long as the infant is gaining weight, this is normal. In the second or third month of life, breast-fed babies may only pass one to two stools a week! As long as the stools are soft, this is nothing to be concerned about.

Bottle-fed babies

Bottle-fed babies tend to have fewer stools than those who are breast-fed and their stools tend to be firmer in consistency.

Straining, grunting, and groaning during a bowel movement

Many infants appear to have trouble passing a stool and grunt and groan, strain and grimace, and go red in the face while attempting to have a bowel movement. They may seem to be uncomfortable, and appear relieved after the stool is passed. Usually the stool is soft and of normal consistency. This is normal, and the difficulty passing the stool is probably related to poor bowel-muscle coordination. This is **not** constipation.

You may sometimes feel it is necessary to aid your infant by rectal stimulation. Do this by using a well-lubricated rectal thermometer or by using infant glycerin suppositories, but these techniques should not be overused. This apparent difficulty with passing stools tends to resolve by three months of age.

Consistency of the stool

The consistency of the stool is more important than the frequency of the stools. **Hard stools indicate a problem.** Constipation is the passing of hard stools (which are often small and pebble-like), and you should discuss this with your child's doctor. The number of stools or frequency of stools does not necessarily define constipation. An infant may be constipated even if he or she is passing several stools a day, and an infant who passes only one stool a week may not be constipated.

Initial treatment for constipation in the first few weeks of life may be to offer the infant one to two ounces of water once or twice a day, or to give diluted juice once or twice a day. Diluted prune or pear juice is often very effective in relieving constipation. If the juice or extra water does not help with the constipation, try rectal stimulation and/or infant glycerin suppositories.

For additional information about constipation, see section on constipation ("To poop or not to poop", page 283).

When to Contact a Physician

- If there is blood in the stools. (A common cause for blood in the stools is a little tear in the anus. This is known as a fissure.)
- If the stools remain hard despite trying the above measures.

Urination.

In the newborn infant the urine may be concentrated (dark) until feeding is well established. When the urine dries on the diaper, it quite frequently has a pinkish color to it. This is not due to blood in the urine but to the presence of urates. The number of wet diapers will give you some indication of how your infant's fluid intake (feeding) is going. Most infants pass urine four to six times a day.

Infections, fevers, and exposure to the outside world

Newborn infants are especially prone to infections because of an underdeveloped and immature immune system. You may decrease your infant's chances of developing an infection by limiting his or her exposure to the outside world. Infections are usually acquired from other people.

- It is especially important to limit your infant's contact with people who have infections such as coughs, colds, and diarrhea.

- Insist that people wash their hands before you let them touch or pick up your infant.
- Do not expose your infant to large crowds of people in shopping malls, churches, and other gatherings in the first two to three months of life.

Fever

If your infant develops a fever (defined as a rectal temperature greater than 100.3° Fahrenheit), you should seek medical attention. **Any fever in the first three months of life needs to be discussed with your child's physician.**

Note: An infant does *not* have to have a fever to be ill. The way that your infant is acting and feeding is more important than the height of the fever. If your infant seems unduly lethargic, sleepy, or is reluctant to feed, contact his doctor.

For further details on fever, see section on fever.

Crying

All babies cry—even healthy babies cry! Many infants cry for up to two hours a day, which is normal. Some infants cry for three or four hours a day, and even this may still be normal for them; such infants are often called colicky.

Babies cry for many reasons—hunger, fatigue, perhaps because they are wet or dirty or just have some vague bodily discomfort. Often we don't know why babies cry; they may just be extra sensitive to their environment.

Colic typically occurs in the evening when babies often have fussy periods. Colicky infants seem to be in pain, cry, and are frequently inconsolable for three to four hours at a time, but the rest of the day the infant is usually content and well. No one knows what causes colic, and the treatment of it is beyond the scope of this book. After a week or two, you will recognize your infant's typical pattern of crying.

Change in type of crying or length of crying

If there is a change in the character of your baby's cry, or if your normally content infant starts crying a lot more, then you should try to find out the cause. Check your infant's temperature. Your child may be in pain (see section on pain), or may be developing an illness.

Your reactions to a crying child

An infant's cry is designed to get attention. Repeated crying often exhausts the parents and leaves them feeling tired, angry, and inadequate.

- If you feel you cannot cope with or tolerate your baby's crying you should seek help urgently. It is natural for a new parent to feel helpless and even resentful at times.

- Try to remember that the crying is not your fault and it is not your baby's fault. You **do** need a break from your infant.

- If you cannot cope and there is no help at hand, just leave you baby in his crib, close the door, and give yourself "time out." Phone a relative, a friend, or your child's doctor.

Never shake an infant! If you should lose control and shake your infant, seek medical care **immediately so that permanent brain damage does not occur,** and explain to the doctor exactly what happened.

FEVER

- Fever is common in childhood and usually occurs in response to an infection, most of which are harmless viral infections.
- Young children get from six to ten infections a year. Each infection may cause a fever for three to four days, so fevers are a common part of growing up!
- Fever is the body's normal response to infection, and activates the body's immune system to help fight the infection. Many experts feel that fever helps your body fight infection. In other words, fever may be your friend and not your foe!
- **If your child has a fever, her behavior is a more important indication of how ill she is than the temperature read on the thermometer.**

Normal temperature ranges.

A child's temperature will vary slightly with age, time of day, and activity. **A child has a fever if the rectal temperature is equal to or higher than 100.4° Farenheit (38° Celsius),** the oral temperature is higher than 99.5° Farenheit (37.5° Celsius) or the axillary (armpit) temperature is higher than 99 degrees Farenheit (37.2° Celsius).

High fevers.

- Most high fevers (greater than 104° Fahrenheit or 40° Celsius) in children are due to harmless viral infections. Parents often worry that a high temperature will cause brain damage. It is extremely unlikely that temperatures below 106° Fahrenheit (41.1° Celsius) would cause brain damage. However, a high fever may be an indication of a serious medical problem which needs attention. See caution below.

CAUTION

Temperatures greater than 106° Fahrenheit (41.1° Celsius) may be due to heat stress caused by over-bundling a child who already has a fever, leaving a child in a hot car, or exercising on a hot day. **Heat stroke** and **heat exhaustion** are extremely dangerous and should be treated immediately (see section entitled "Heat Related Illness", page 384.)

• Unless your child is over-bundled or confined to a heated environment, or exercising excessively, the fever does **not** continue to go up and up. Before the temperature reaches 106° Fahrenheit, the body's thermostat will reset the temperature to a lower level and the fever will drop one to two degrees or more. If your child is over-clothed or swaddled in blankets, the fever could continue to rise to dangerous levels. So keep your child **lightly dressed!**

Your child's behavior.

• **How a child acts is far more important than the height of the fever.** A child with a temperature of 104° Fahrenheit who is alert and active may be less ill than a child with a temperature of 101° Fahrenheit who is extremely lethargic and not showing any interest in the surroundings.

- Many children with a fever are lethargic and irritable. Some children with a high fever may be confused and may even hallucinate. They often breathe faster than usual. However, once the fever is reduced, your child should perk up and be more alert. He may even have periods of playfulness. The breathing rate should return to normal. **If your child is not acting normally once the fever is brought down, then you should contact a doctor because the underlying illness may be serious and require treatment.**

- The height of the fever does not necessarily correlate with the severity of the illness. A simple viral infection, which is not at all serious, may cause a temperature of 104° Fahrenheit or higher, whereas a serious bacterial infection that may require urgent therapy, may only cause a fever of 102° Fahrenheit or lower.

- Seizures: Four percent of children may develop a short convulsion with a fever. This is known as a febrile convulsion and does **not** cause brain damage, although it may age the parent! Your doctor should be notified because the cause of the fever should be identified. (See section on Convulsions, page 289.)

How to take your child's temperature

- A child's temperature may be taken with a glass thermometer (oral or rectal), a digital thermometer, or an ear thermometer. Digital thermometers are much easier and quicker to use than glass thermometers and are much cheaper than ear thermometers. Temperature-sensitive strips are not very accurate.

CAUTION

Glass thermometers may contain mercury, which is extremely poisonous. This is a serious hazard if a thermometer is broken.

- Before using a glass thermometer, remember to shake it down well. It should be left in the rectum for at least two minutes, in the mouth for 3 minutes, or under the arm for four minutes.

- **A rectal temperature is the only reliable way to measure a temperature in the first three months of life.**

- Ear temperatures are acceptable, except in the first three to six months of life when they may be less accurate.

Rectal Temperature.

Place your child on your lap, lying on his stomach.

Lubricate the thermometer tip using Vaseline or KY jelly.

Gently insert the tip into the rectum about one inch. Hold it in place for two minutes if using a glass thermometer. A digital thermometer will beep when it is time to read the temperature.

Remove the thermometer and wash it.

Oral Temperature.

Make sure your child has not had hot or cold food or drinks within the past thirty minutes.

Slide the clean thermometer alongside and under the tongue.

Hold the thermometer in place and make sure the mouth remains closed.

If using a glass thermometer, remove and read the temperature after three minutes.

A digital thermometer will beep when the temperature has been recorded.

Underarm Temperatures.

Place the thermometer tip in a dry armpit.

Hold the arm against the chest for four minutes if using a glass thermometer.

A digital thermometer will beep when ready to be read.

How to treat your child's fever.

1. Clothing and environment

- When your child has a fever, keep her lightly dressed—ideally she should be stripped down to a diaper or underpants.
- If your child shivers, cover her with a light, cotton blanket or cotton T-shirt.
- Keep your child's room comfortably cool.

2. Fluids

- Encourage your child to drink extra fluids. Give small amounts of liquids frequently.
- If your child is nauseous or vomiting, let her suck on ice chips.

3. Medicines

- **Never** use aspirin to treat fever in a child. It may cause a serious illness known as Reye's Syndrome.

- Use fever-reducing medication (acetaminophen or ibuprofen) if your child is uncomfortable and the temperature is higher than 102° Fahrenheit (38.9° Celsius). Both medications are extremely safe if used appropriately.

- Unless your child's temperature is only mildly elevated, **neither acetaminophen nor ibuprofen will return your child's temperature to normal.** They will only reduce the fever by two or three degrees, for example from 104° Fahrenheit to 102° Fahrenheit.

- **Neither medication will work if your child is over-bundled or over-clothed!**

- You may need to dose these medications repeatedly because their effects will wear off after a specified number of hours, and the fever will continue to go up and down as the illness runs its course.

- **Give the correct dose of the medication.** If you underdose, the medication may not be effective; if you overdose, there is an increased risk of side effects. Refer to the manufacturers recommendations and to the section "A children's medical kit."

- Do not continue either medication for longer than three or four days without consulting your child's doctor. Long-term use of acetaminophen may cause liver damage and ibuprofen may cause stomach upset, stomach bleeding, and kidney damage.

- Some experts feel it is better **not** to treat a fever as it is helping the body fight the infection!

ACETAMINOPHEN

Acetaminophen is available as infant drops, children's suspension, chewable tablets, tablets, and suppositories.

- To administer the infant drops, **use the infant dropper supplied with the medication.**
- **Many over-the-counter medications contain acetaminophen.** This applies particularly to cold medications. Check that these do not contain acetaminophen as **it is very easy to over-dose your child if you are using several different medications.**
- The temperature-lowering effects of acetaminophen usually last three to four hours.

IBUPROFEN

Ibuprofen is available as infant drops, children's suspension, chewable tablets and tablets.

- To administer the infant drops, **use the infant dropper supplied with the medication.**
- Ibuprofen is longer-acting and its effects usually last six to eight hours.
- Ibuprofen is **not** approved for use in the first six months of life.

4. Sponging
- Combine sponging with medication.
- Unless your child cannot tolerate acetaminophen and ibuprofen, give a dose of one of these medications first.
- **Never** put alcohol in the water.

YOU MAY WANT TO SPONGE YOUR CHILD WITH LUKE-WARM (NOT COLD) WATER IF:

- Your child's temperature is higher than 104° Fahrenheit (40° Celsius).
- Your child has had seizures during past fevers.

- Your child is confused and refuses to take medication by mouth (acetaminophen suppositories would be an alternative).

- Your child is vomiting and can't keep oral medication down (acetaminophen suppositories would be an alternative).

- Your child is allergic to acetaminophen and ibuprofen.

WHEN TO SEEK MEDICAL CARE

It is extremely difficult to give hard-and-fast guidelines when one is talking about fevers in children. A child who has a relatively low fever may have a serious cause for the fever which requires early and expert medical care. On the other hand, a child with a high fever may just have minor viral illness and not require any special care.

Generally speaking, the younger the child, the more seriously you should take the fever. This definitely applies to the first three months of life and to a lesser extent to the first two years of life. Some experts feel that any child in the first two years of life who has a fever lasting longer than twenty-four hours **without any obvious cause** (such as a cold, earache, sore throat, diarrhea, etc.) should be seen by a physician.

Guidelines to help you decide when to seek medical care:

- If your child is less than 3 months of age and has a rectal temperature equal to or above 100.4° Farenheit (38° Celsius).

- If your child is excessively lethargic, drowsy, or has other worrying symptoms such as abdominal pain, severe headache, neck stiffness, rapidly-spreading rashes, and repeated vomiting and diarrhea.

(continued)

WHEN TO SEEK MEDICAL CARE *(continued)*

- If your child still looks very ill after the temperature has been brought down to below 100.4° Farenheit (38° Celsius).

- If your child has a fever that lasts longer than three to four days.

- If your child has a seizure. If your child has a short seizure and is acting normally after the seizure, it may not be necessary to see a physician, but it is wise to discuss the episode with one.

- Anyone developing a fever while in a malarial area, or after visiting a malarial area, may have malaria. Consult a physician. Malaria has an incubation period of at least seven days, so if your child gets a fever within the first week of visiting a malarial area, it is unlikely to be due to malaria. (See section on malaria.)

Remember, how your child acts is more important than the height of the fever!

TREAT YOUR CHILD, NOT THE FEVER!

If, despite reading the above guidelines, you're still concerned about your child's condition, seek medical care. **There is no substitute for getting your child assessed by a competent medical professional.**

PAIN

Pain is a common symptom of many childhood illnesses and is discussed in more detail with the various causes of pain, for example, earache under "Ears and Flying" and "Ear Infections," belly ache under "Abdominal Pain," and head pain under "Headache." Each section contains guidelines about when to seek medical attention.

Generally, if pain continues for more than three to six hours or is unresponsive or poorly responsive to a mild analgesic (such as ibuprofen or acetaminophen), then medical attention should be sought. Seek medical care earlier if your child is in severe pain. If other symptoms, such as breathing difficulties, are also present, you should seek help immediately.

It is especially difficult to determine the cause and severity of pain in children in the first three years of life because they have trouble vocalizing their symptoms and localizing pain. Pulling and tugging on the ears in a young child often is due to teething or perhaps your child has just "discovered" his ears! This rarely indicates an ear infection.

In children of any age symptoms may be misleading, as pain is often referred from one part of the body to another. A child with pneumonia may complain of bellyache and a child with a hip problem may complain of knee pain.

When assessing a young child who is fussy and seems to be in pain, it is important to undress the child completely and examine him or her closely for the cause.

Rash

Are you able to see any rashes? Non-blanching rashes, which spread rapidly, may be a sign of a serious infection. Blanching is determined by applying pressure to the rash with a fingertip to check if the rash fades.

Lumps or swelling

Can you detect any lumps or swellings? A lump in the groin may indicate a hernia, and a swelling in the scrotum may indicate a strangulated testicle.

Belly

Is the abdomen distended? Does your child cry or resist when you push on his abdomen? Sit your child on your lap and distract him by telling a story or reading a book while you feel his abdomen.

Fingers and toes

Always check fingers and toes carefully. A thread of cotton or a piece of hair may have become entwined around a finger or toe and be cutting off circulation.

Arms and legs

If you move your child's limbs, does he cry out in pain? If your child has learned to walk, get him to walk. Watch how he moves his arms and legs. A child who refuses to stand or walk may have a painful hip (for example, from a hip infection) or a fractured leg (which may be caused by a seemingly minor fall or injury). On the other hand, the child may have a serious abdominal condition such as appendicitis. Children with severe belly pain will usually refuse to hop and if asked to walk will often walk bent over.

Medications

Is your child on any medication? Many cough and cold medications may make children fussy and inconsolable. Some antibiotics, for example erythromycin, may cause severe abdominal pain.

When to Consult a Physician

It is always preferable to discuss your child's pain and any other worrying symptoms with a medically qualified person. If you are traveling this is not always possible. Even an experienced pediatrician may have difficulty in determining the cause of fussiness or pain in a young child. A child who appears to be severely ill may have a relatively minor cause for his symptoms such as colic or an earache while another child who does not appear that ill may have a ruptured appendix! If your child is older than six months, it is acceptable to administer an appropriate dose of acetaminophen or ibuprofen and see if this settles your child. **If, despite administration of an analgesic, pain or fussiness persists, then medical attention should be sought.**

If there are other symptoms or findings present such as breathing difficulties, repeated vomiting, cold extremities, or non-blanching rashes, seek medical care immediately.

COLDS, UPPER RESPIRATORY INFECTIONS (URI'S), "RUNNY NOSE," AND NASAL CONGESTION

In the first few years of life, most healthy children get between five and ten colds a year! This is a normal part of growing up and does not mean that your child has something wrong with his immune system.

A typical cold in a young child lasts about ten days. It usually begins with a low grade fever (99–102° Fahrenheit), nasal congestion, clear nasal discharge and fussiness. Usually within two to three days, the fever will settle and the nasal discharge will turn yellowish or green and become thicker. This colored nasal discharge will last for five to eight days before becoming clear again and then will disappear. Often your child will have a loose cough which is worse when lying down, on waking up, or when active. The cough may persist for a week or so after the cold has disappeared and is usually more prominent in the evening.

Treatment.

Colds are viral infections and will **not** respond to antibiotics. In other words, **antibiotics should <u>not</u> be taken for a cold.** There are no wonder medications for colds and nothing will turn a ten-day cold into a five-day cold!

There are a number of things you can do to make your child more comfortable:

- Encourage your child to drink fluids. This **includes** your child's normal formula or milk.

- Use a cool-mist humidifier in the room at night. This will moisten your child's mucous membranes and help to get rid of the mucus. **The humidifier should be discontinued once the cold is over.**

- If your child has a fever or is very fussy, it may be worth trying a dose of acetaminophen (*Tylenol*). This may relieve some of the discomfort.

- Over-the-counter cough and cold medicines make very little difference and may make the nasal secretions thicker. They may also make your child fussy and irritable. It is preferable **not** to use these during the first six months of life.

- If your child's cough is very troubling, try giving your child *Benadryl* in the evening before she goes to bed. This will **not** get rid of the cough but may decrease it.

- If your baby has trouble feeding or breathing and the nasal secretions are very thick, administer nasal saline (salt-water) drops into one nostril at a time and aspirate the mucus with a bulb syringe. Your infant or child will not appreciate this but it often opens up the nasal passages. It is especially helpful to do this just prior to feeding. Nasal saline drops are extremely safe and may be purchased over the counter or made up at home by dissolving ½ level teaspoon of salt to 8 ounces of water.

- Nasal decongestant drops, such as ¼% ephedrine nose drops, are often very effective in relieving nasal congestion but should **never** be used for longer than four to five days continuously. Do **not** exceed the recommended dose. These drops can also have very unpleasant side effects.

REASONS TO SEEK MEDICAL CARE

1. Lethargy, extreme fussiness, or refusal to take liquids.

2. Your child appears sicker than you would expect from a simple viral cold.

3. Your child complains of severe earache or severe headache. (A young child or infant is not able to vocalize symptoms and may just be very fussy.)

4. A rectal temperature above 100.3° Fahrenheit in an infant **in the first three months of life.**

5. If your child has symptoms suggestive of a complicating bacterial sinusitis:

   • A fever that lasts longer than four to five days.

   • A colored nasal discharge persists beyond fourteen days.

   • A day-time cough that lasts longer than fourteen days.

   • Your child is sicker than you would expect from a cold:

     — The fever is above 103° F.

     — Your child has a severe headache or facial pain.

     — Extreme irritability or lethargy.

6. Your child or infant seems to have trouble breathing. Many young infants and children have a lot of trouble breathing when they have a cold. If this does not improve after suctioning of the nose, seek medical care. (See also section on Breathing Difficulties.)

Notes:

- Just because your child has a yellowish-green nasal discharge does **not** mean your child has bacterial sinusitis and needs an antibiotic.

- If you are traveling and you are concerned your child may have an ear infection as well as a cold but you do not have access to medical care, do not despair—**eighty percent of ear infections will resolve without antibiotic treatment.** (See section on ear infections, page 231.)

- If your child has a persistent, foul-smelling discharge from just one nostril you should suspect a foreign body in the nose and have your child seen by a doctor.

- Allergies are usually the cause of a prolonged clear and watery discharge from both nostrils.

SORE THROAT

A sore throat (pharyngitis or tonsillitis) is common in childhood and is usually due to a viral infection, although strep (a bacterium) is also a common cause of a sore throat.

A **viral sore throat** does **not** respond to antibiotic treatment, so antibiotics should **not** be used with one. The pain and fever will **not** go away any faster if an antibiotic is used. Viral sore throats are often accompanied by a cold or a runny nose, a cough, and hoarseness. They tend to come on gradually.

Strep throats are rare below the age of one year. Usually someone with a strep throat does not have a runny nose or cough. A child with strep throat will often appear ill and sometimes have a headache, abdominal pain, and swollen and tender glands in the neck. Another clue that the sore throat may be due to strep is a faint reddish rash that is usually more noticeable in the groin, armpits, and elbow creases. Strep throats often come on suddenly and sometimes there is a history of contact with someone with strep.

A child with a strep **or** viral sore throat may have a fever and white spots may be seen on the tonsils. The presence of white spots on the tonsils does **not** necessarily mean "strep." The **only reliable way** to tell the difference between a viral sore throat and a strep throat is with a rapid strep test or a throat culture.

A fairly common cause of a viral sore throat in a young (six months to four years) child is herpangina (hand, foot, and mouth disease). A child with this illness tends to be very unhappy, is often drooling excessively, and may have a high fever. Sometimes there is diarrhea and a rash. If you can get a good look at the back of your child's mouth, you may see shallow ulcers. This is a viral illness and antibiotics are **not** indicated and not helpful.

228 ◆ PEDIATRIC HEALTH PROBLEMS

Treatment.

Neither viral nor strep throat is a medical emergency. Strep throat does not have to be treated right away!

Home treatment consists of giving analgesics (acetaminophen or ibuprofen) and drinking fluids. Sucking on ice pops or ice chips is often soothing. An older child (six years of age and over) may be helped by sucking on lozenges or gargling with salt water. (Mix half a level teaspoon of salt in 8 oz. of water).

Antibiotics are indicated for strep throats but not for viral sore throats. One of the hallmarks of a strep throat is that the patient improves rapidly (usually within twenty-four hours) after antibiotics are started.

When to consult with a physician.

If you suspect strep throat, have your child seen by a medical professional within two to three days. Most strep throats will get better even without an antibiotic—the symptoms just take longer to go away.

The main reason antibiotics are used to treat strep throat is to prevent the later development of rheumatic fever. This is fortunately very rare in the United States. Studies indicate that as long as the antibiotics are started within nine days of the onset of the illness, rheumatic fever should be averted. The other reasons antibiotics are used to treat strep throat are to limit the spread of the infection and to make the patient feel better sooner. If you are traveling and do not have access to medical care, then symptomatic care may be sufficient.

Remember, four out of five sore throats are due to viruses and do not require antibiotic treatment!

Please help your child's doctor to practice good medicine by not insisting an antibiotic be prescribed for probable viral illnesses—colds, most sore throats, and bronchitis.

DISTINGUISHING BETWEEN VIRAL AND STREP SORE THROATS

VIRAL	STREP
Frequency	
Very common, accounts for 80 percent of sore throats	Common, but less common than viral sore throats
Age	
Any	Rare in the first year of life. Not common in the second year of life
History of strep contact	
Not usually present	Often present
Onset	
Often gradual	Frequently sudden
Fever	
May or may not be present	Almost always present
Other features	
Nasal congestion, cough, and hoarseness often present	May have headache and abdominal pain, typical strep rash, and/or enlarged and tender neck glands

(Continued on next page)

DISTINGUISHING BETWEEN VIRAL
AND STREP SORE THROATS
(Continued from previous page)

VIRAL   **STREP**

Throat findings

May have white spots on   May have white spots on
tonsils   tonsils. Throat often a beefy
                                red color. May have minute
                                red spots on the hard and
                                soft palate

Treatment

Analgesics and fluids   **Antibiotics,** analgesics,
                                and fluids

Response to Antibiotic

None   Rapidly gets better on
                                antibiotics

Note: There is a great deal of overlap between the symptoms and signs of viral and strep sore throats. The **only** reliable way to tell them apart is with a throat culture or a rapid strep test. Neither cause of sore throat is a medical emergency.

EARACHE AND EAR INFECTIONS

There are two common types of ear infection:

- **Middle ear** infection (otitis media).
- **Outer ear infection** (otitis externa, also know as "swimmer's ear").

It is common to have ear pain with both of these infections. Many young children complain of earache, even in the absence of ear disease. The apparent earache is commonly due to other causes such as teething or a sore throat. **Pulling or tugging on the ear is a very unreliable sign of ear disease in infants and young children and does not mean necessarily that an ear infection is present.** Children above three to four years of age can usually report accurately when they have an earache.

A) OTITIS MEDIA/MIDDLE EAR INFECTION

Infection of the middle ear is the most common type of ear infection and the most common cause of ear pain. It is particularly common in infants and young children and is usually associated with a cold or upper respiratory tract infection. The pain is often worse when the child is lying down.

Common symptoms are fever and fussiness, the latter often being worse at night. The symptoms of the associated viral URI (upper respiratory tract infection), such as nasal stuffiness often are more impressive. Some children have no apparent symptoms at all and the ear infection is discovered incidentally at a routine medical examination!

Treatment

Treatment consists of:

- **Analgesics** (usually acetaminophen or ibuprofen) in adequate doses.
- **Antibiotics.** Despite the fact that antibiotics are usually prescribed for middle ear infections, **the majority of middle ear infections will get better without antibiotics.** In many countries antibiotics are not routinely prescribed for ear infections. However, the infection and symptoms will usually resolve faster with antibiotics.

  Antibiotics should probably be used if:

  — your child is less than two years of age

  — your child has a fever above 102° F

  — your child has severe earache

  — your child's symptoms last longer than 2 to 3 days

Sometimes the eardrum perforates due to pressure behind the drum and blood-stained pus may discharge from the ear canal. Although this is often alarming to parents, this is not an emergency, and the pain should immediately lessen. The eardrum will usually heal on its own within a few days but you should follow up with your child's doctor to check that it has healed completely.

At times a child will wake in the middle of the night with a severe earache. This may be helped with an **appropriate** dose of acetaminophen or ibuprofen, by propping up the head of the bed so that the child's head is elevated, and by instilling warm oil drops (such as olive oil) in the affected ear. Do **not** put oil drops in the affected ear if it is already perforated or if your child has had tubes inserted. Middle ear infections are not contagious but the cold that leads to the ear infection is contagious.

B) OTITIS EXTERNA OR "SWIMMER'S EAR"

Swimmer's ear is more common in older children. It is more common during the summer months, as this the time they are usually swimming. This is an infection of the ear canal which leads from the outer ear to the eardrum.

Symptoms include earache, a sense of fullness in the ear and often itching. The pain is increased if the ear lobe is pulled or pressure is applied to the tab covering the opening of the ear canal. At times the pain may be very severe.

Treatment

This consists of:

- Analgesics, as listed for otitis media.
- Eardrops, either over the counter or prescription. Sometimes oral antibiotics are needed as well. If the pain persists beyond twenty-four to forty-eight hours despite treatment, or is very severe, your child should be seen by a physician.

While your child has swimmer's ear, he should **not** submerge his head when swimming. Try to keep his ears as dry as possible.

Prevention of swimmer's ear

Swimmer's ear tends to be recurrent and prevention is extremely important. Keep the ears as dry as possible:

- After swimming, have your child shake his head and jump up and down to get rid of excess water in the ears.
- Dry the ears carefully and gently, using a Q-tip.
- Administer eardrops to prevent otitis externa. These may be purchased over the counter or made by mixing

equal quantities of rubbing alcohol and white vinegar. This homemade preparation will sting if the ear canal is already inflamed. Do **not** use these drops if your child's eardrum is perforated or tympanostomy tubes are in place.

COUGH

- A cough is a common symptom in childhood.
- The most common cause of a cough is a cold.
- A cough is a protective reflex and ejects foreign material and secretions from the airway.
- A cough is called "chronic" if it lasts longer than three weeks.
- Coughs often disturb the parent more than the child!

There are many different types of coughs, and even more causes of coughs. The following are some of the more common causes of coughing in children.

The cold cough.

The cough associated with the common cold is typically a loose, "junky" cough. It lasts for the duration of the cold (seven to ten days) and often for one week afterwards. The cough will occur on and off throughout the day, but is usually more severe in the early evening and in the first hour or two after going to bed.

The cough tends to subside in the middle of the night, but as soon as your child awakens and stands up in the morning, the cough will return and be more severe for an hour or two. Frequently, the mucus is swallowed and then vomited up later.

When you hold your child his chest may feel "rattly" and you may think that the cold is in the chest or that he has pneumonia. The rattle that you are feeling is the vibration and gurgling of the mucus in the back of the throat that is being transmitted to the chest. If your child is not in respiratory distress (breathing very fast or retracting) when the coughing bouts are over, then it is less likely that he has pneumonia. For discussion on retracting and assessment of respiratory distress, see section on breathing difficulties, page 409.

During coughing bouts, your child may become red in the face, and may even seem to be choking on the mucus. This is common and will settle when the mucus is swallowed or coughed up or vomited.

It is common for a child to have five to seven colds a year, so it is quite possible that he may cough for ten to fourteen weeks a year! Many colds occur back-to-back resulting in coughs that appear to last for three to five weeks. This makes recurrent colds the commonest cause of a chronic cough!

Treatment

A cough associated with a cold usually does not require specific treatment.

- It is important to keep your child well hydrated.

- Using a cool mist humidifier in the room at night for a week or two may help. **The humidifier should be discontinued once the cold has resolved.**

- If the cough is extremely troublesome, then an appropriate dose of *Benadryl* may help to suppress the cough. There are many other cough medicines on the market, and ones containing dextromethorphan are usually safe and fairly effective in childhood.

- In young infants, using nasal saline drops and a bulb aspirator is often very useful in keeping the nose clear and so enabling your child to breathe more easily.

Sinusitis and coughing.

Sinusitis is also a very common cause of coughing. The features of a sinusitis cough are often very similar to those of the cough associated with a cold: the cough occurs when lying down, and often has a loose, "junky" quality. However, with sinusitis, the cough tends to be more troublesome during the daytime and usually persists for longer.

Often there is not much drainage out of the nose, and you may think that the mucus that your child coughs up is coming from the lungs. However, with sinusitis the mucus usually drains from the sinuses and down the back of the throat. The cough reflex is then triggered, and the mucus comes back out through the mouth.

Symptoms that suggest your child's cough has turned into bacterial sinusitis are the duration of the cough (longer than ten to fourteen days) and a persistent daytime cough. The color of the mucus is not helpful in identifying sinusitis, because it tends to be yellow or green with both a viral cold and sinusitis. Facial pain or painful teeth are sometimes present in older children and adults with bacterial sinusitis.

Treatment

A sinus cough will respond to an appropriate antibiotic, but it may take a week or two for the antibiotic to relieve the symptoms. Additional medications that may be necessary include oral antihistamines and decongestants, decongestant nose drops and occasionally a nasal steroid spray may be prescribed.

Like ear infections, most cases of sinusitis will resolve without antibiotics but the symptoms may persist longer.

Persistent severe headache, a persistent fever or tenderness over the forehead or cheek bones definitely indicate a visit to a doctor.

Croup and coughing.

Croup and stridor should be taken seriously because they can cause a child's airway to close suddenly!

Croup is usually due to a viral infection of the upper respiratory tract and mainly affects the voice box (vocal cords) and windpipe (trachea). It often comes on very suddenly in the evening or at night. With croup, your child may have a barky cough and make a raspy noise (stridor) when breathing in. The airway narrows with croup and this may lead to severe breathing difficulty. This can be very frightening for both the child and parent. Your child's voice will also probably be hoarse.

Both the barky cough and the stridor are usually worse at night. As dawn approaches, they tend to lessen, only to return the next evening. The barky cough and stridor will often last up to a week, but with each successive night the cough and stridor should lessen.

Treatment

- A croupy cough is often helped by humidification of the air. Use a cool mist humidifier in your child's bedroom at night. Do **not** continue to use the humidifier once your child's croup has resolved (usually five to seven days).

- If the cough and stridor worsen, take your child into the bathroom and turn on the hot taps and steam up the bathroom. Sit there with your child for fifteen minutes.

- If your child still has a severe cough and stridor, then going outside and breathing in the cool night air for five to ten minutes may bring relief. If this does not help, seek medical attention.
- Sleep in the same room as your child because croup can get worse rapidly (See section on breathing difficulties.)
- If your child turns blue, passes out, or stops breathing, call 911 immediately. Start CPR if necessary.

Allergies and cough.

Allergies may cause a cough from a post-nasal drip, irritation of the upper airway, or by triggering asthma. If the trigger is allergy to house dust mites the symptoms may be worse at night and hoarseness is sometimes present in the morning. Often nasal stuffiness is present as well.

Treatment

An allergic cough will respond to removal of the trigger and to the administration of an antihistamine such as *Benadryl* or one of the newer, non-sedating antihistamines. Nasal steroid sprays and occasionally oral steroids may be needed.

Asthma.

Asthma is probably the second most common cause of a chronic cough in childhood. It tends to be worse in the middle of the night (12 AM to 3 PM) and after exercise.

> **NOTE:**
>
> Your child does not have to
> wheeze to have asthma!

A child who has recently had a cold and continues to cough between 12 AM and 3 AM for several weeks **after** the cold has run its course, often has asthma. In contrast, the cough associated with a cold usually only lasts two to three weeks.

A child with asthma often has had eczema in the past and frequently other family members have allergic diseases such as allergic rhinitis and hayfever.

There are many triggers for asthma such as upper respiratory tract infections, cold air, exercise, allergies, and irritants such as cigarette smoke. Exercise in cold air is a particularly potent trigger for an asthmatic cough.

Treatment

An asthma cough will respond to appropriate asthma medications. These should include a preventative/controller drug, as well as a "rescue" drug. It is also essential to identify and avoid asthma triggers (See section on asthma.).

"Irritation" cough.

An "irritation" cough is often started by a viral infection, but then the cough continues to be triggered once the underlying viral infection has resolved. Triggers include cigarette smoke, perfumes, paint fumes, smoke from fires and stoves, and cold air.

This type of cough tends to be dry and does not produce mucus.

Treatment

Remove the trigger. Humidifying the air and sucking on cough lozenges or cough suppressants often help. Keep your child away from cigarette smoke!

Beware of foreign bodies!

If your child starts coughing after choking on food, he may have inhaled some food. This is particularly likely when eating foods such as peanuts, raisins, and hot dogs. Your child may also inhale foreign bodies such as small toys and beads.

Treatment

If you suspect your child has inhaled a foreign body, seek medical attention immediately. (See section on choking, page 414.)

Coughs while traveling.

It is not unusual to develop a cough while traveling. Causes may include

- The dry air of the aircraft cabin.
- Exposure to cigarette smoke, noxious fumes, and so on.
- The development of an upper respiratory tract infection (a cold).
- Activation of preexisting asthma.
- If it develops while you are at a high altitude, a cough may be a sign of high altitude sickness. (See section on altitude sickness, page 157.)
- A chest infection, such as bronchitis or pneumonia.

Several types of cough at the same time

Many children have more than one cause of a cough and more than one type of cough at any one time. For example, an asthmatic child with a cold may have a loose, "junky" cough in the evening when he first lies down, followed by a tight cough between midnight and 3 AM. As he awakens in the morning, the loose, "junky" cough returns. Later on that day, the asthmatic child will often cough with exercise. Children with asthma frequently have nasal allergies and sinusitis as well. They are also more likely to have gastro-esophageal reflux (regurgitation of stomach contents up the esophagus).

A child with a cold or postnasal drip will often cough more with exercise.

Children exposed to cigarette smoke cough more than other children. **Exposure to cigarette smoke makes all coughs worse and makes them last longer.**

WHEN TO CALL OR VISIT YOUR CHILD'S DOCTOR

- Signs of respiratory distress such as breathing very fast, retractions, etc. (See section on breathing difficulties).
- You suspect an inhaled foreign body.
- Any cough that lasts longer than three weeks.
- A cough during the first few months of life.

In summary, by far the most common cause for a cough is a cold. **Remember, coughs are often there for protection.** They stop the mucus from going down into the chest.

NOSEBLEEDS

Nosebleeds occur frequently in children and have many causes. The most common cause is nose picking. Other causes include colds, allergies, sinusitis, and exposure to very dry air, especially in heated homes in winter. Nosebleeds are very common at high altitudes due to the dry and cold air.

When you suction your infant's nose with a bulb aspirator a small amount of bleeding may occur.

Treatment of a nosebleed.

- Have your child sit up, lean forward, and breathe through the mouth.
- Pinch the soft fleshy part of the nose tightly closed for about ten minutes.
- Hold a basin under the chin to catch any blood or mucus that drips through the mouth. After the nosebleed has stopped, instruct your child not to pick his nose or to blow it too vigorously, otherwise the bleeding may restart.

Prevention

- If the air in your home is too dry, use a humidifier and **try to keep the humidity around forty percent.** Remember, if your house or bedroom has high humidity for prolonged periods, you will encourage the growth of molds and replication of house dust mites, which in turn may lead to allergies.
- Use salt water (saline) nose drops frequently while traveling. The dry air of the aircraft cabin and dusty air while traveling on country roads will lead to a dry and

stuffy nose. Each person should have his or her own bottle of saline drops!

- If your child has repeated nosebleeds, coat the lower part of the nasal septum (the part of the nose dividing each nostril) twice a day with a *Vaseline*-type petroleum jelly.

- Discourage nose picking! Stopping nose picking is not a very easy thing to do!

WHEN TO SEEK MEDICAL CARE

- If your child's nose continues to bleed after applying pressure to the nose for twenty minutes. (If you do not have access to medical care and you have nasal decongestant nose drops such as *neosynephrine* or *Afrin,* use these, as they constrict blood vessels and will often help to stop the nosebleed. **Never use nasal decongestant drops or sprays for longer than five days.**)

- If your child has a foul smelling or bloody discharge from one nostril for some days. This may be due to a foreign body up the nose.

- If your child has a tendency to bleed in other areas as well, for example from the gums or into the skin.

- If your child gets recurrent nosebleeds despite using preventive measures.

SOME COMMON EYE PROBLEMS IN CHILDREN

Eye problems in children are a common cause for concern to parents and a frequent reason to visit the doctor. Discussed below are some of the more common eye problems seen during childhood.

"Pink eye."

When parents, teachers, and daycare providers talk of "pink eye"they usually are referring to an infection involving the conjunctiva, the transparent outermost covering of the front of the eye and the inner eyelid. The correct medical term for this type of "pink eye" is infectious conjunctivitis. It is important to realize that there are many other causes of pink or red eyes besides infectious conjunctivitis. Some of these causes are far more serious than the usual "pink eye."

Important causes of pink or red eyes

- **Inflammation of the conjunctiva (conjunctivitis).**
    - **Infectious conjunctivitis** is the most common cause of "pink eye" and is discussed in detail below.
    - **Allergies. Allergic conjunctivitis** is more common in people who tend to get allergies. It usually involves both eyes and is very itchy. If an eye discharge is present it is usually clear. Common triggers are pollens and cats.
    - **Chemicals and Irritants.** Chemicals and irritants may also cause red eyes. Common causes are shampoos, soap and chlorine. Most people can remember

getting red and sore eyes after swimming in an over-chlorinated swimming pool! One may also get red and irritated eyes when exposed to a smoky environment.

- **Inflammation of the cornea (keratitis).** The cornea is the clear part of the eye in front of the pupil (the dark spot in the center of the eye) and the iris (the colored part of the eye).
- **Inflammation of the iris (iritis).**
- **Raised pressure within the eye (glaucoma).**
- **Eye injuries.**
- **Foreign bodies.**
- **Tumors.**

Infectious conjunctivitis (usual "pink eye")

This is the most common cause of "pink eye." This type of "pink eye" is contagious. It may be caused by viruses, bacteria, or a combination of the two. Children with infectious conjunctivitis usually have red eyes and often an eye discharge. Sometimes the child may be sicker and have a fever as well as other symptoms such as sore throat or earache. Teachers and daycare personnel are frequently more concerned about the contagiousness and possibility of spread to other children than the "pink eyes" of the infected child! Parents are not only concerned about their child but also the days that they will have to take off work while their child is excluded from daycare or school!

It is often very difficult to differentiate between "pink eye" caused by bacteria, which responds quickly and dramatically to antibacterial eye drops or ointment, from "pink eye" caused by viruses which usually gets better more slowly and often without any specific treatment.

DIFFERENCES BETWEEN BACTERIAL AND VIRAL CONJUNCTIVITIS

	Bacterial	**Viral**
Age:	Usually younger (average three-and-a-half years).	Usually older (average eight-and-a-half years).
Eye Discharge:	Usually thick and "goopy". Often yellow or green. Eyes often glued together in the morning.	Usually thinner and more watery.
Associated Illnesses:	May also have an ear infection.	May also have a sore throat.

In practice there is so much overlap between bacterial and viral conjunctivitis that it may be impossible to tell the difference between the two. This is one of the reasons why both are usually treated with antibacterial eye drops or ointment. Sometimes antibiotics by mouth are needed as well. Most daycares and schools will allow your child back once he has been on treatment for twenty-four hours.

TREATMENT OF INFECTIOUS CONJUNCTIVITIS (PINK EYE)

1. Hygiene. Infectious conjunctivitis is very contagious!

— Wash your hands well after touching your child's eyes and after instilling eye drops or ointment into the eyes.

— Wash your child's hands frequently.

— Use a separate washcloth and towel for your child.

— Avoid kissing your child on the face while he has conjunctivitis.

— Do not share utensils or food while your child is infected.

2. Topical medication.

— These include eye drops and eye ointments.

— Eye drops are generally easier to instill. Ointments are often prescribed for infants. Treatment is usually prescribed three times a day. Twice a day may be sufficient if some of the newer preparations are used. These are very fast-acting and effective.

— The duration of treatment will depend on the cause, the severity, and the response to treatment and will usually be from three to seven days. **It is usually a good idea to continue the treatment for a day or two after the eye discharge has cleared.**

— It is easier to instill the medication if you first clean away the eye discharge with a wet cotton ball.

— Putting eye drops or eye ointment in the eyes of young children can be quite a challenge! Fortunately most of the newer preparations do not sting but despite this you may need two well-coordinated adults to instill the medication. If your child refuses to open his eyes, put two drops of the medication in the corner of his eye while he is lying down. When he opens his eyes the drops will go in.

3. Oral antibiotics. These are often prescribed for associated ear infections. They are also used alone for uncooperative children who resist topical medication. They seldom work as fast as topical treatment.

If you have no access to medical care or medication, it may be reassuring to know that most cases of infectious conjunctivitis will get better on their own but just take longer to do so. Even the ear infection that is often associated with infectious conjunctivitis frequently resolves on its own!

Bathing the eyes with cotton balls soaked in clean water or in a weak salt solution (½ tsp. table salt to 1 cup water) will soothe the eyes and help clear away the discharge.

NOTES:

- Do not use contact lenses when the eyes are infected!
- Never put steroid eye drops or steroid ointment in the eyes without an eye doctor's advice.

As mentioned above there are many other causes of "pink eye." Parents who are away from home and do not have easy access to medical care will need to know when they really do need to get medical help.

EYE PROBLEMS—WARNING SIGNS AND SYMPTOMS—REASONS TO SEEK MEDICAL CARE EARLIER OR IMMEDIATELY.

— **Pain.** Most cases of infectious "pink eye" are associated with mild discomfort. Viral conjunctivitis often gives one the sensation of a foreign body in the eye. **Severe eye pain warrants immediate medical attention.** In young children who are unable to vocalize their pain, crying or extreme irritability may be an indication that they are in pain.

— **Blurred vision or loss of vision.** Any difficulty seeing should be taken very seriously. Sometimes a large amount of pus in the eye will cause blurry vision, but once this is wiped away the vision should be normal. Eye ointments may also cause blurry vision. This is one of the reasons why it is preferable to use eye drops rather than ointment when treating anyone older than one year of age.

— **Severe light sensitivity (photophobia).** This often indicates corneal involvement.

(Continued on next page)

EYE PROBLEMS—WARNING SIGNS AND SYMPTOMS—REASONS TO SEEK MEDICAL CARE EARLIER OR IMMEDIATELY.

(Continued from previous page)

— **Trauma.** Any history of eye injury is of concern.

— **Foreign body.** Seek treatment if you think there is a possibility that your child may have something in her eye. As mentioned above, viral conjunctivitis may give a foreign body sensation in the affected eye.

— **Irregular pupils.** If you notice that the black spot in the center of the eye (the pupil), is irregular.

— **The pupils are not of equal size.**

— **The cornea is cloudy.**

— **Increasing redness with treatment.** This suggests your child may be allergic to the eye drops or ointment!

— **Persistence of "pink eye."** Most cases of infectious conjunctivitis begin improving within twenty-four hours of starting treatment and are much improved after forty-eight to seventy-two hours of treatment. In contrast, some cases of viral conjunctivitis take many days to get better. Let your doctor decide why your child is not getting better!

— **Marked swelling around the eye.** This may indicate an infection of the skin and underlying tissues (cellulitis) or sinusitis.

— **Pink eye that only involves one eye.** Although bacterial and viral conjunctivitis may start in only one eye, usually within a day or two they have spread to the other eye as well.

— **Blisters involving the surrounding skin.**

MORE SERIOUS CAUSES OF INFECTIOUS CONJUNCTIVITIS:

Herpes conjunctivitis. The same virus that causes "cold sores" can cause "pink eye." Clues to herpes conjunctivitis are:

- Only one eye is involved.
- Severe pain.
- Blisters surrounding the eye.
- Impaired vision.
- Contact with "cold sores."

However, none of these clues may be present, the person may have herpes conjunctivitis! In other words, herpes conjunctivitis may look identical to other, less serious causes of "pink eye." Specialized treatment is required to preserve the vision.

Conjunctivitis in the newborn. Sticky eyes are commonly seen in the newborn infant (see below) and are not serious. However, occasionally newborn babies may have very serious causes for conjunctivitis. These usually present with very pussy and swollen eyes and immediate and expert treatment is necessary.

As mentioned at the beginning of this section, there are other causes of "pink eye" besides inflammation of the conjunctiva. These include many serious causes such as inflammation of the cornea (keratitis), raised pressure within the eye (glaucoma), eye tumors and trauma. **The eyes are delicate structures. Don't delay in seeking medical advice or treatment!**

Eye Concerns in the Newborn Infant

1. Red marks in the newborn's eye

Many newborn infants have red, flame-shaped marks in the white part of the eyes. These are hemorrhages that occurred during delivery. They are of no concern and fade over the ensuing 2 to 3 weeks. No treatment is necessary.

2. Yellow eyes

The whites of many newborns eyes turn yellow in the first few days of life. This is known as jaundice and is extremely common in the first week or two of life. Your baby should be checked by a medical professional **in the first week of life** to make sure the jaundice is not severe. Often your child's bilirubin level will be checked. Occasionally your baby will need treatment (phototherapy lights) to lower the bilirubin level.

3. "Sticky" eyes

Many babies develop slightly "sticky" eyes. You may notice a discharge from one or both eyes. This is often more marked in the morning and after naps. Usually the whites of the eyes are nice and clear. Despite treatment, this "stickiness" or discharge tends to recur. This is frequently due to blocked tear ducts which may involve one or both eyes. The tear ducts usually open spontaneously sometime during the first year of life. Occasionally surgery is required to open a blocked tear duct. This is usually done in the second year of life.

4. Newborn conjunctivitis

Newborn infants may also develop infectious conjunctivitis and is most often caused by bacteria. One or both eyes will be pussy and red. Your child's doctor may want to prescribe antibiotic treatment. **If your child's eyes are very swollen and pus is pouring out from**

between the eyelids, immediate treatment needs to be instituted. If not treated aggressively, permanent eye damage may result!

Styes.

A stye is a small abscess on the margin of the eyelid. It may be very irritating but is not usually serious. Treatment consists of warm compresses many times a day. Often antibiotic eye drops or ointment is prescribed as well. They frequently take days to weeks to resolve.

Eye injuries.

Trauma is one of the more important causes of vision loss in childhood. Boys are more commonly involved than girls. Boys between 11 and 15 years of age are particularly at risk.

➤ Corneal abrasions

These are the most common eye injury. Your child will complain of severe eye pain as well as be light sensitive and have tearing. Your child needs to be seen by a doctor who, after examining the eye, will probably prescribe antibiotic eye ointment or drops as well as pain medication. Patching of the eye used to be standard treatment but is now infrequently done.

➤ Foreign bodies

These most frequently involve the conjunctiva or cornea. Objects commonly involved are specks of dirt, pieces of grass, hairs, and similar objects. Try the following to get rid of the foreign body:

— Blinking.

— Specks of dirt may sometimes be removed by lifting the upper eyelid up and outward and drawing it down over the lower lid.

— Try to wipe out the foreign body using a clean tissue or Q-tip.

— Flush it out of the eye using an eye wash.

If none of the above methods work, seek medical attention. **Do not rub the eye.**

Occasionally specks of metal may penetrate deep into the eye. This should be suspected when working around metal.

Never attempt to remove objects embedded in the eye. Seek medical attention.

➤ Sports injuries and blows to the eye

These can result in bleeding within the eye and you may see blood layering within the eye. If you observe this or there is reduced vision or severe pain, seek medical attention immediately. Apply cold compresses without excess pressure to help reduce pain and swelling. Do not use ibuprofen (*Advil* or *Motrin*) as an analgesic as this may increase the tendency to bleed.

➤ Lacerations and punctures of the eye

Do **not** try to wash out the eye with water and do **not** instill any eye drops or ointment. Do **not** try to remove any object protruding from the eye. Cover the eye with a cut-off paper or polystyrene cup and seek medical attention immediately.

Burns of the eye

These may be caused by:

— **Hot objects.** Cigarette burns of the cornea are not uncommon in children. The affected part of the eye often has a white appearance. Medical attention should be sought. Fortunately the eye often heals without scarring.

   Burns from fireworks are usually far more serious and often result in the loss of vision. (See section on fireworks injuries, page 400.)

— **Chemicals.** Both acids and alkalis can lead to very severe eye injuries. These are true medical emergencies! Alkali burns are far more dangerous than acid burns and tend to penetrate deeply. Alkalis that are commonly found around the home include ammonia, bleach, drain openers, cleaning solutions, fertilizers, lime and cement. **Immediate** treatment should be instituted. This should consist of **copious irrigation** of the eye using running water or pouring water into the eye from a clean container. This irrigation should continue for thirty minutes. This should also help remove any particulate matter. **Seek medical attention.**

Prevention of eye injuries

Most eye injuries are preventable.

— Store chemicals safely, out of reach of children.

— If you regularly handle chemicals, have an eye wash station readily available.

— Wear goggles when using jumper cables or handling acids, alkalis, strong cleaning fluids and chemical sprays.

— Don't allow young children to handle scissors, sharp pencils, and similarly dangerous objects.

— Teach your child not to run with sharp objects in his hands.

— Do not let your child play with pellet guns, darts, and similar dangerous missiles.

— When you mow the lawn, make sure your child is a safe distance away. Stones can be thrown for many yards by power mowers.

— When working with power tools, wear eye goggles.

— When teaching your child how to hammer nails, make him wear goggles.

— Never allow your child to play with fireworks. Keep a safe distance away when other people are lighting fireworks. Bystanders are frequently injured by bottle rockets.

— Wear protective eye guards or spectacles when playing contact sports or sports involving ball "missiles" such as baseball and racquetball.

— When fishing, make sure your child is a safe distance from you. Fishing hooks can be very dangerous.

— Be careful when opening champagne bottles. Their corks may become very dangerous missiles!

— Respect the sun. Wear sunglasses. Never look directly at the sun or at an eclipse of the sun.

VOMITING, DIARRHEA, AND DEHYDRATION

See also: Section on travelers' diarrhea, page 102.
Section on vomiting, page 257.

AN OVERVIEW

Definition of diarrhea.

Causes of vomiting and diarrhea.

How to recognize dehydration . . . table

Management of vomiting and diarrhea.

- Treating mild illness with no dehydration
    In the first year of life.
    In children older than one year
- Treating mild and moderate dehydration.
- Treating severe dehydration.

More on fluid therapy, appropriate solids and vomiting.

- Electrolyte solutions
- Other acceptable fluids
- Liquids to be avoided
- Foods
- Vomiting

Medications to treat diarrhea and vomiting.

Miscellaneous.

- Stools
- Weight loss
- Hygiene

When to seek medical attention.

Summary.

Appendix A.

Definition of diarrhea.

Diarrhea is defined as the increase in the frequency and looseness of bowel motions.

Causes of vomiting and diarrhea.

There are many causes of diarrhea and vomiting in infants and children. Most cases of acute diarrhea are due to an infection of the bowel (gastroenteritis), most commonly caused by a virus. **Viral gastroenteritis** usually occurs in the winter months and often begins with a fever and vomiting. Diarrhea usually develops later. Most normal infants and children get occasional bouts of viral gastroenteritis. Younger children tend to be more severely affected.

Other causes of diarrhea:

- Bacterial diarrhea. This tends to be a summer illness. The stools may contain mucus and blood. Sometimes antibiotics are needed to treat this.

- Travelers' diarrhea is usually caused by bacteria.

- A breastfed infant often has frequent loose or watery stools, but in the strict sense of the definition this stool pattern should not really be classified as diarrhea as it is the infant's normal state. This is no cause for concern if the infant is active and gaining weight. If you notice that your infant's stool pattern is changing (for example, larger, more watery stools or a change in odor) or your infant's behavior is changing (for example, your infant is more irritable or more lethargic) then you should discuss this with your child's physician.

- Excessive consumption of juice may cause diarrhea.
- Sometimes diarrhea and vomiting are symptoms of another disease such as a urinary tract infection, meningitis, or appendicitis. If your child looks ill, is lethargic, or has severe pain, he should be seen by a physician.

No matter what the cause of diarrhea, an important goal is to prevent and treat dehydration. Children become dehydrated because of a loss of fluids and electrolytes (salts) from vomiting or diarrhea, or a combination of the two. This dehydration is further compounded by inadequate fluid and food intake.

Even in the United States, dehydration caused by vomiting and diarrhea is a significant cause of hospitalization and death! As with travelers' diarrhea, **the younger the child, the greater the likelihood of becoming dehydrated.** Older children and adults tolerate fluid and electrolyte losses better than infants.

How to recognize dehydration.

A child's behavior is a very sensitive sign of the degree of illness. A child who is lethargic, lying around, and showing no interest in the environment is probably significantly ill. An alert child who is interacting with his environment and crawling or running around is probably not significantly ill or dehydrated.

Refer to the table that follows.

Factors Used to Assess Dehydration	Signs and Symptoms		
	Mild Dehydration	Moderate Dehydration	Severe Dehydration
Mental status and activity level	Normal: alert and interactive	May be normal but usually listless, less active, and irritable	Lethargic (apathetic, sluggish, very little interest in surroundings, drowsy)
			May be weak, floppy and limp.
			May be comatose
Thirst	Slightly increased	Moderately increased	Very thirsty or too ill and lethargic to indicate thirst
Mucous membranes of mouth	Slightly dry	Dry Tongue will have a sandpapery feel	Very dry
Tears	Present	Absent	Absent
Eyes	Normal	Sunken	Very sunken
Fontanel (soft spot)	Normal (a slight depression of the soft spot is normal)	Sunken	Very sunken
Urine output	Slightly decreased and a little darker (more concentrated)	Decreased, very dark (very concentrated)	Very little to no urine, very dark
Severe dehydration is a medical emergency and requires _immediate_ medical attention.			Additional signs of severe dehydration include: • Cool and mottled extremities • Very weak pulses • Tenting of the skin: if the skin on the abdomen or chest is pinched up, it stays up for a short while

Management of vomiting and diarrhea.

Your goal is to prevent dehydration by giving extra fluids <u>as soon</u> as the vomiting and diarrhea starts.
Using the table immediately above, classify your child according to his state of hydration:

- No dehydration.
- Mild dehydration.
- Moderate dehydration.
- Severe dehydration

And then follow the guidelines below . . .

❖ Treating *mild* illness with *no* dehydration

- Your goal is to **prevent** dehydration. To do this your child will need to drink **extra** fluids to replace the fluids that are lost. It is usually only necessary for your child to **drink more of the liquids he usually drinks.**

➢ IN THE FIRST YEAR OF LIFE

- Continue your child's usual feedings, either breast or formula. **Offer these feeds more frequently.**
- **If the diarrhea increases in severity,** give other fluids such as water and electrolyte solutions (*Kaolectrolyte, Pedialyte, Infalyte, Liquilyte, Ceralyte*). Children of this age will usually drink electrolyte solutions despite their salty taste. Special electrolyte solutions such as those mentioned above are **not** essential in managing **mild**

diarrhea in a child who is **not** dehydrated. Other fluids that can be given include diluted juices (one-third strength) or sports drinks such as *Gatorade* (half strength). *Liquilyte* is the best tasting of the ready made electrolyte solutions.

- If your child is eating solids, appropriate foods to offer are cereals such as rice cereal and oatmeal, mashed potatoes, and mashed bananas.
- *Avoid* full-strength juice, sodas, and *Jello.*

VOMITING:

- A breast-fed baby may be able to continue to breast-feed if fed for **shorter periods** and **more frequently**.
- If your child vomits more than two to three times, discontinue milk feeds and **offer small amounts (1 teaspoon)** of clear fluids (such as those mentioned above) every one to two minutes. This is a full-time job but may save your child a hospital admission.
- After a couple of hours try to reintroduce milk feeds in **small** quantities. Give frequently. If these are retained, offer the recommended solids.
- If your child continues to vomit or shows any signs of dehydration, seek medical help.

➢ CHILDREN OLDER THAN ONE YEAR

- Unless your child is vomiting, continue with normal foods and fluids but give more of these fluids.
- If the diarrhea and vomiting increases, give extra fluids such as water, diluted juices (one-third strength) or half strength sports drinks such as *Gatorade*. These are acceptable if given with starchy foods such as cereals, mashed potatoes, saltines, and pretzels.

- **Avoid** full-strength juices, sodas, and *Jello*.
- Continue to offer extra fluids until the diarrhea has resolved.
- If the diarrhea continues to increase in severity, and especially if the stools are large and watery, it is preferable to give electrolyte solutions.

VOMITING:
- If your child vomits more than two to three times, stop milk feeds and solids.
- Offer **small volumes** (1–2 tsp.) of clear fluids such as electrolyte solutions, diluted juices, or diluted *Gatorade* **frequently.**
- Offer your child popsicles or ice chips.
- Seek medical attention if your child continues to vomit or shows signs of moderate to severe dehydration.

❖ Treating *mild* and *moderate* dehydration

If your child is dehydrated she is likely to be more ill and will probably be very thirsty, have a dry tongue and sunken eyes. The more dehydrated she is, the more apathetic and lethargic she will be. The situation is now more serious. Contact your child's physician if possible. However, if you are on the road and don't have access to a physician, don't panic. Most children with mild and moderate dehydration can be successfully rehydrated if you follow the guidelines below. You have your work cut out for you, so settle down, put aside all other activities and devote yourself to getting fluids into your child.

What fluids to give:

Once a child is dehydrated it is preferable to give commercially prepared electrolyte solutions such as *Kaolectrolyte, Infalyte, Pedialyte, Liquilyte,* or *Ceralyte. Liquilyte* is the best tasting of these.

How much fluid to give:

Children who are mildly dehydrated will need to get one ounce of fluid for every pound they weigh. Children who are moderately dehydrated will need to get two ounces of fluid per pound body weight. It is not always that easy to assess the degree of dehydration. Consequently, for practical purposes, you should **aim to give your child about one and a half ounces of fluid per pound body weight over the next four hours.** Adjust the amount you give according to your child's response.

How to give this fluid:

<u>**If your child is vomiting**</u> it is essential to give very small amounts often. Follow these guidelines:

- In children less than thirty or forty pounds (usually two to four years of age)—start by giving one teaspoon every one to two minutes. You may have to use a medicine dropper to do this.

- In children over forty pounds (usually over four years of age)—start by giving two teaspoons every one to two minutes. Try using a medicine cup to give this fluid.

For example, if your child is one year old and weighs about twenty pounds and is mild to moderately dehydrated, she will need to drink about thirty ounces over the next four hours to replace the fluid she has lost. (If you give her one teaspoon (5ml) of fluid every minute, she will get 10 oz. over one hour and 40 oz. over 4 hours!)

Children who are not vomiting may be given much larger volumes of fluid.

After about an hour of giving fluids every minute and once you are sure your child is tolerating these fluids, you may give slightly larger volumes less often.

Extra fluid:

Extra fluid will be required to replace fluid lost by continuing diarrhea and vomiting: For each watery stool in a child less than two years give an additional 4 oz. of fluid. For each watery stool in a child older than two years offer an additional 8 oz. of fluid.

Most vomits do **not** contain a large amount of fluid. However, if you feel your child had a large vomit offer an additional 2–4 oz. fluid, but give this fluid slowly over the next thirty to forty minutes or so.

> *Example:* A ten-month-old who weighs twenty pounds and who is mildly dehydrated will need approximately 20 oz. over the first four hours (1 oz. per pound). If this child passes two watery stools during this four-hour period she will need an additional 8 oz. of fluid for a total of 28 oz.

For practical purposes, many experts recommend giving an extra one ounce of electrolyte solution per pound body weight over the next 8 hours. This is given **in addition** to your child's regular diet of fluids and solids.

- **Reassess your child's level of hydration repeatedly and adjust the volume of fluid to be given accordingly.**

Feeding:

When the dehydration has been corrected, your child's usual diet should be given.

❖ Treating *severe* dehydration

A child who is severely dehydrated will appear very ill. He will be lethargic and floppy and not be interested in his surroundings. He may even be unresponsive and possibly in coma. His eyes will be sunken and he will have a very dry mouth. The tongue will have a leathery feel. He may not be able to drink. Often his hands and feet will be cold and mottled. There will be little or no urine output.

This is a medical emergency and immediate medical attention is required!

More on fluid therapy, appropriate solids, and vomiting

FLUIDS

Types of fluids:

a) Electrolyte solutions

- These are sometimes known as oral rehydration solutions or ORS. Examples of these are *Pedialyte, Kaolectrolyte, WHO-ORS, Liquilyte,* and *Ceralyte.* These are ideal for rehydrating children and adults with dehydration. Of these, **Liquilyte** is the best tasting but only comes ready mixed.

- Some of these electrolyte solutions taste very salty but you can improve the taste by adding 1–2 drops of *NutraSweet* or a little sugar-free *Kool-Aid* powder.

You can also improve the taste by adding 2–3 tsp. of apple or grape juice to every 8 oz. of electrolyte solution. Better tasting, fruit-flavored electrolyte solutions are now commercially available.

- Electrolyte solutions can be frozen and offered as popsicles. Popsicles made from electrolyte solutions are now commercially available. Electrolyte solutions can be made into ice cubes which can be crushed and offered as ice chips.

- Homemade ORS can be used as described in the chapter on travelers' diarrhea, but **it is always better to use commercially ORS** because homemade ORS may not have the correct concentration of salt. Homemade ORS should only be used in emergency situations when commercially made ORS is not available.

- **Most electrolyte solutions do not lessen the severity or duration of the diarrhea.** They just prevent and treat dehydration. Giving solids may lessen the severity and shorten the duration of the diarrhea. *Ceralyte* may also lessen the severity and shorten the duration of diarrhea.

- It is **not** necessary to use electrolyte solutions if your child has only mild diarrhea and is not dehydrated.

The younger the child and the more severe the diarrhea and dehydration, the more important it is to use electrolyte solutions.

b) Other acceptable fluids

- Breast milk is an ideal fluid for most infants. If your infant vomits breast milk, offer the breast more often but let your child feed for **shorter periods**.

- Formula may be offered if your child is not vomiting and is well hydrated. Again, smaller feeds given more often may be better tolerated. Stop the formula if your infant is vomiting. Try and reintroduce the formula four to six hours later.

- Do not dilute milk or formula unless your child is vomiting, and even then dilute it only for **short** periods. When you dilute milk or formula you also dilute the calories!

- Some infants and children are unable to tolerate milk or formula because of temporary sugar (lactose) intolerance. Lactose intolerance may be present if your child passes a large watery stool after each milk feed. These infants and children should be given a lactose-free preparation such as soy milk (*Isomil, Isomil DF, ProSobee*) or lactose-free milk (*Lactofree, Lactaid Milk*). Older children do not need milk at this time.

- Vegetable juices such as carrot juice.

- Diluted fruit juices or sodas (one-third strength), half strength *Gatorade* or water may be used for **short** periods, in mild to moderate diarrhea, and especially if supplemented with **starchy** and **salty foods** such as rice cereal, oatmeal, mashed potatoes, and mashed bananas in a young child. Older children and adults should eat salted crackers or pretzels to increase the fluid and salt absorption.

c) Liquids to be avoided

- Full strength fruit juices, sodas, sports drinks, and *Jello* should **NOT** be given unless these are the only fluids you have available! They have a very high sugar content and no or insufficient salts. **They frequently make the diarrhea worse!**

- Most commercial chicken broth has too much salt and no sugar so it is **not** suitable for rehydration.
- Do **not** give boiled skim milk.

YOUR CHILD'S USUAL FOOD

- Do **not** starve your child. Cooked cereal such as oatmeal or cream of wheat, mashed potatoes, rice, noodles, wheat (such as bread, saltines, crackers, and pretzels), and bananas will aid in water absorption, will shorten the period of diarrhea, and decrease its severity. Lean meats, yogurt, vegetables, and fruit are usually well tolerated. Bananas are a good source of potassium which is lost in diarrheal stools.
- **Avoid** fried and fatty foods.
- **Avoid** foods which contain a lot of sugar such as ice cream and *Jello*.
- If your child is vomiting or is dehydrated, you should stop his normal diet for a period of four to six hours. Slowly try to reintroduce appropriate fluids and later, solid foods.
- The "BRAT" diet (bananas, rice, applesauce and toast) may be acceptable to use for **short** periods (one to two days) but does **not** supply enough calories, protein, and fat for long-term use.

VOMITING

- **Vomiting is NOT a contraindication to giving electrolyte solutions.** Even infants and young children who are vomiting will usually be able to tolerate **small** volumes of electrolyte solutions. **Give 1 tsp. (5 ml.) every one to two minutes.** In older children, you may use a medicine cup. As the fluid is tolerated, increase the volumes and give less often.

- Children above eighteen months of age may suck on ice chips or popsicles if vomiting is a problem. Electrolyte solutions may be made into popsicles which your child can suck on, or into ice blocks, which can then be crushed and offered as ice chips.

- Breast-fed infants who vomit should be fed for shorter periods and more often.

- If your child continues to vomit despite these measures, then medical care should be sought.

Medications to treat diarrhea and vomiting

Antibiotics

Antibiotics make most cases of diarrhea worse and are usually not indicated. However, occasionally they may be needed, for example in some cases of bacterial diarrhea and travelers' diarrhea.

Anti-motility agents

These agents slow the progress of food through your child's intestinal tract. These include loperamide (*Imodium AD*) and diphenoxylate hydrochloride (*Lomotil*).

- *Lomotil* should **never** be given to treat childhood diarrhea.

- *Imodium AD* may be used in older children and adults who do not have a high fever, abdominal distention, or blood in their stools. *Imodium AD* is often helpful in older children and adults with travelers' diarrhea. **However, this should not take the place of giving fluids by mouth.** For the dosages and side effects of *Imodium*. See travelers' disease, page 32.

Agents to firm the stools

Agents such as *Kaopectate* may firm the stools, but they do not shorten the illness and may detract from the primary purpose of giving fluids by mouth. It is preferable **not** to use such agents.

Bismuth subsalicylate (*Pepto Bismol*)

Pepto Bismol has been shown to be effective in preventing and treating travelers' diarrhea. It is seldom indicated in the management of non-travelers' diarrhea in children, even though it has been shown to decrease the frequency of unformed stools. There are side effects and contraindications to using *Pepto Bismol* (see section on travelers' diarrhea).

Medications to stop vomiting (anti-emetics)

It is usually **not** advisable to use these medications in children because they may have very unpleasant side effects.

Miscellaneous

ABOUT STOOLS

- Contact your child's physician if there is blood in the stool.
- Stool color is not important. When your child has diarrhea, the stool color may vary from brown to yellow to bright green, but this should be of no concern. Many medications and fluids may change the color of the stools.
- *Pepto Bismol* may turn your child's tongue and stools black.

- Do not be concerned if you see pieces of food in your child's stool.
- The amount of fluid lost with each stool will depend on the age of the child, the size of the stool, and its consistency. Replace each watery stool in a child less than two years of age with 4 oz. of electrolyte solution and each watery stool in a child older than two years of age with 8 oz. of electrolyte solution. At times large watery stools may contain more than 8 oz. of fluid.

ABOUT WEIGHT LOSS

The *initial* cause of weight loss in a child with gastroenteritis is dehydration. However, a common cause for weight loss *later* in the illness, especially if your child is well hydrated, is starvation! In other words, your child has not been given the essential nutrients to maintain and gain weight. Children usually regain this once they are eating normally.

HYGIENE

Remember to wash your hands well after changing your child's diaper.

Dispose of disposal diapers in a hygienic and environmentally-friendly way.

WHEN TO SEEK MEDICAL ATTENTION

Consult with your physician:

- If your child is less than six months old and has diarrhea or vomiting.

- If your child is limp and lethargic, or appears very ill.

- If your child has any signs of dehydration. It may not always to be possible to contact a medical professional while traveling. However, if you follow the guidelines above, you should be able to rehydrate your child on your own.

- If your child has vomiting that persists despite the measures described above and the dehydration is worsening. In most children the vomiting settles on the second day of the illness.

- If your child refuses to take liquids by mouth.

- If your child has a severe stomach ache lasting longer than two hours. Note, however, that many children have recurrent bouts of abdominal pain or cramps, especially when passing gas or stools. Persisting pain (longer than one or two hours) or worsening pain indicates the need to seek medical attention to rule out more serious causes of pain such as appendicitis, bowel perforation, obstruction, etc.

- If the stool contains a large amount of mucus or blood, or is black (and your child is not taking *Pepto Bismol*).

- If the diarrhea is not *improving* after three to four days. It may take as long as seven to ten days before your child's stools are totally normal, but each day there should be improvement. Your child should be eating and drinking well, and be active, alert, and interested in his or her surroundings.

SUMMARY OF THE MANAGEMENT OF VOMITING AND DIARRHEA

1. **Give extra fluids as soon as the vomiting and diarrhea starts**—do **not** wait for your child to become dehydrated.

2. Give **appropriate** fluids by mouth:
   - Give generous amounts unless your child is vomiting.
   - Give small amounts often if your child is vomiting.

3. **Avoid** fluids and foods that may make the diarrhea worse.

4. **Feed** your child solids unless your child is vomiting or dehydrated.

5. **Continue giving extra fluids until the diarrhea has resolved.**

Appendix A

Conversion of pounds (lbs.) to kilograms (kgs.):

Approx. 2 lbs. equals 1 kg.

Conversion of ounces (oz.) and quarts to milliliters (ml.) and liters (l.):

Approx 1 oz. equals 30 ml.

Approx. 1 quart equals 1 liter.

VOMITING

See also: Section on Vomiting, Diarrhea, and Dehydration, page 257.

Just as there are many causes for diarrhea, abdominal pain, and fever in childhood, there are many causes for vomiting in childhood. Some of these are serious, but most are of no concern unless the vomiting is repetitive and accompanied by other symptoms.

- Many infants spit up or regurgitate small amounts of milk or food in the first year of life. This is normal and usually totally harmless. It may lead to a high laundry bill but does **not** usually lead to dehydration! This repeated regurgitation is known as **gastro-esophageal reflux** (GER). If your child is not gaining weight adequately, or is always fussy, or has breathing problems, he may need to be treated. Otherwise, you just need to wait until your child has outgrown this, which usually happens around one year of age.

- **Projectile vomiting** in the first three months of life often has a significant medical cause and if it occurs repeatedly you should seek medical attention. In projectile vomiting the vomited material "shoots out" many feet.

- In the first few weeks of life an infant who vomits green colored fluid may have a bowel obstruction and needs to be seen by a medical doctor urgently.

- The sudden onset of vomiting in the older infant or child is most often due to an **acute gastroenteritis,** usually caused by a viral infection of the bowel. The vomiting usually lasts one to two days, and is often accompanied by a fever. Diarrhea frequently develops later. The major concern here is the same as with diarrhea—your child may become **dehydrated**. (See section on diarrhea and dehydration.)

- It is important to remember that there are **other serious causes of vomiting** such as appendicitis or other medical conditions (for example, meningitis or a kidney infection) which require urgent medical care.

Treatment of vomiting

The treatment of vomiting varies according to the cause.

Below are some guidelines to help you prevent your child from becoming dehydrated. (See also the section on diarrhea and dehydration.)

— All solids and milk products (apart from breast milk) should be stopped for four to six hours.

— Give **small** amounts of clear fluids to your child.

In a child under one year of age, it is usually best to give oral rehydration solutions (ORS). In older children, sips of water or diluted *Kool-Aid* or *Gatorade* or similar fluid may be given as long as the vomiting does not continue beyond six to twelve hours. Sucking on ice chips made from *Liquilyte* or some other electrolyte solution is also a good way to get fluids into a vomiting child.

One cannot stress enough that the secret to success is giving small amounts (as little as a teaspoon or a medicine dropper full) frequently. Your child may be thirsty and will probably want to drink a full bottle or full glass of liquid but this will almost certainly lead to vomiting.

— Increase the volume of fluid offered once the smaller volumes are tolerated.

— After four to six hours of clear fluids and with no vomiting, it is usually safe to reintroduce formula to a younger infant or a bland diet to the older child. This may consist of saltine crackers, rice, mashed potatoes, bananas, etc.

It is important **not** to starve your child for prolonged periods but **to get him back on a normal diet as quickly as possible.**

What about medications to stop vomiting?

These frequently have unpleasant side effects in children and should only be used under the direction of your child's doctor.

REASONS TO SEEK MEDICAL CARE

- Vomiting that persists beyond twenty-four hours in a child less than two years of age, and beyond forty-eight hours in a child over two years of age. You may need to seek medical attention earlier, especially in young children and if the vomiting is severe or repetitive.

- If your child develops signs of dehydration such as a dry mouth, sunken eyes, or lethargy. (See section on diarrhea and dehydration.)

- Projectile vomiting in the first year of life. Every child is allowed to have the occasional projectile vomit, but if this happens repeatedly, medical care should be sought.

- Your child appears unduly ill or is lethargic and apathetic. In other words, your child's condition appears to be worse than can be explained by the degree of vomiting.

(Continued on next page)

REASONS TO SEEK MEDICAL CARE
(Continued from previous page)

- Bile-stained vomiting (yellow or green vomit) in the first six months of life or persistent bile-stained vomiting in older children.

- If there is a large amount of blood (more than a teaspoon), or blood clots in the vomit and your child has not just had a nosebleed. There may be streaks of blood in the vomit if your child retches repeatedly.

- If your child has severe abdominal pain. Children who vomit will be unhappy and uncomfortable, but they should not be in severe pain once each vomiting episode is over.

- If there is a swelling in the groin (this may be a hernia or a strangulated testicle).

- If your child has obvious abdominal distension (the abdomen appears very full).

- If your child has other worrying symptoms, such as severe headache, neck stiffness, confusion, or backache.

- If your child's condition is worsening.

STOMACHACHE/BELLYACHE/ ABDOMINAL PAIN

• There are many causes of stomachache in children varying from such simple causes as indigestion or gas pains to serious causes such as appendicitis and obstruction of the bowel.

• Remember, children below two to three years of age have trouble localizing pain. They may complain of bellyache when in fact they have a middle ear infection or some other illness.

• Sometimes the pain may not even be due to an abdominal condition but be due to referred pain from a chest condition such as pneumonia.

Common causes of abdominal pain in childhood.

1. **Constipation.** This is probably the most common cause of abdominal pain in childhood! (See section on constipation, page 283.)

2. **Strep throat.** This is a particularly frequent cause of bellyache in the school age child. (See section on sore throat/ URIs/strep throat, page 223.)

3. **Dietary "indiscretion."** This includes eating too fast, eating too much, and eating food that does not "agree" with one! Many children with lactose intolerance get stomach cramps and diarrhea when they eat dairy products. This condition often runs in families.

4. **Acute gastroenteritis.** This often begins with abdominal pain. Vomiting, fever, and diarrhea usually follow soon afterwards. (See sections on vomiting, page 275, and diarrhea and dehydration, page 257.)

5. **Infantile colic.** (See section on the newborn infant, page 199.)

6. **Emotional upset.** Many children get a tummy ache when they are upset or worried. Anxiety related to problems at school or home is common.

Abdominal pain or stomach upsets while traveling may be due to a combination of factors: constipation, dietary indiscretion, and the anxiety associated with travel. It may also be the first sign of travelers' diarrhea!

Other more serious but far less common causes of abdominal pain include urinary tract infections, appendicitis, intestinal obstruction, poisoning, and many, many other causes.

Management of bellyache.

Fortunately, most bellyaches disappear on their own.

The treatment of abdominal pain will obviously depend on the cause. Initially the cause of the pain may not be obvious and so one usually tries to comfort a child with a caring and commonsense approach. Below are some guidelines:

- Encourage your child to lie quietly and rest. During bouts of abdominal pain, reassure your child in a calm voice and tell him to take a few deep and slow breaths.

- If the pain persists, try a warm water bottle or a heating pad on your child's belly.

- Sucking on ice chips may help to distract your child as well as maintain hydration.

- Do **not** give your child medicines that may confuse the situation or make matters worse. Avoid aspirin- and ibuprofen-containing products. Unfortunately acetaminophen (*Tylenol*) rarely helps belly ache. Sometimes a dose of *Pepto Bismol* or *Maalox* may help relieve the pain.

Before you call your child's doctor, consider the following:

If:

- The cause is constipation; follow the guidelines in the section on constipation. Encourage your child to sit on the toilet and to try and have a bowel movement. **Tackle the problem of constipation because unless it is dealt with properly and diligently it is sure to come back again!**
- The cause is lactose intolerance; avoid lactose-containing foods such as milk and cheese. Discuss this further with your child's doctor at your next routine visit.
- You suspect strep throat, seek medical care.
- It becomes obvious that the bellyache was the harbinger of acute gastroenteritis; follow the guidelines in the section on vomiting, diarrhea, and dehydration.

REASONS TO SEEK MEDICAL CARE

- The pain increases in severity or lasts longer than three to six hours.

- Your child has repeated vomiting.

- Your child has signs of dehydration. (See section on dehydration.)

- Your child is unable to walk or walks bent over. Many children with appendicitis walk bent over, move very gingerly, and are reluctant to hop.

- Your child is persistently tender over the appendix area (lower right side).

- Your child vomits blood.

- Your child has blood in the bowel movements.

- Your child vomits bile (green or yellow fluid).

- Your child has a swelling in the groin or swollen and painful testicles.

- Your child has recently had an abdominal injury.

- Your child appears very ill, has a high fever (greater than 104° F), is very pale, has cold or mottled extremities, or is confused or is very lethargic.

- You suspect your child has strep throat. (Not a medical emergency!)

Happily, most children with a bellyache are not seriously ill. Your child will get better and you will have a few more grey hairs! Discuss the pain with your child's doctor. Hopefully you can prevent a recurrence.

TO POOP OR NOT TO POOP: CONSTIPATION AND OTHER BOWEL PECULIARITIES

Definition of constipation.

When defining constipation one needs to take three things into account:

a) The consistency of the stools.

b) The frequency of the stools.

c) The difficulty in passing stools.

There are many definitions of constipation but a commonly accepted one is the **passage of hard stools** often accompanied by **pain**. Some definitions might include the word "infrequent" but this is not always the case. A person may only pass a stool once or twice a week but if the stool is soft and not accompanied by discomfort then one would not label that person as constipated. This is often the case in breast fed infants in the second and third months of life.

A) The first year of life

THE CHANGE IN A CHILD'S BOWEL HABITS WITH AGE AND DIET

• In the first few days of life infants pass meconium stools. These are black and tarry but within two to five days the stools are usually yellow or green or various shades in between. Sometimes the stools have a seedy texture.

- Typically, a **breast-fed infant** will have frequent (as many as five to ten) stools a day, and these stools are often loose or even watery. Despite this, the infant is content, gaining weight and thriving. Frequently, around the second or third month of life, breast-fed babies only pass one to two stools per week! As long as the stools are soft and the infant is content and gaining weight this is regarded as normal. This infant is **not** constipated and does not require any treatment!

- **Formula-fed infants** usually have far fewer stools a day and the stools tend to be firmer and more smelly. If the stools are hard and the infant appears to be in pain when passing them, one would say the infant is constipated and treat the infant accordingly. This is more likely to occur if the infant is on soy feeds.

Apparent difficulty in passing stools: Many infants in the first few months of life appear to have great difficulty passing in stools. They get red in the face, strain, grunt, cry, draw their legs up over the abdomen . . . and eventually pass a totally normal, **soft** stool! This is normal and is probably due to immature coordination of the muscles of the bowel. As long as the stool is soft and the infant is otherwise well and thriving, this is nothing to be concerned about. This problem usually resolves by three to four months of age. Such an infant is **not** labeled as constipated. Imagine how difficult it must be to poop while lying on your back!

MANAGEMENT OF STOOLING PROBLEMS IN THE FIRST YEAR OF LIFE

First of all ask yourself if your baby truly is constipated or is it just a bowel coordination problem? If the latter, then no treatment may be the best treatment! If you feel your infant really does need help, try stimulating the rectum by inserting a well lubricated (*Vaseline* or *KY* jelly) thermometer about 1 inch into your infant's rectum. Alternatively, insert an infant glycerine suppository into your infant's rectum. Usually within a few minutes a stool will be passed. Although effective, these techniques should not be overused!

If your infant has **true constipation,** there are a number of things you can try:

- Offer your infant an ounce of water once or twice a day.
- Give your infant an ounce of prune or pear juice diluted with an equal volume of water once or twice a day.
- Add 1–2 tsp. of dark *Karo* syrup to your infant's formula once or twice a day.
- Consider using the infant glycerine suppositories described above.
- If your infant is already eating solids, add baby foods high in fiber such as apricots, pears, prunes, peaches, peas, and beans.

If the above measures fail, consult your child's doctor. A **medical examination** and **prescription stool softeners** may be indicated.

B) Constipation in toddlers

Toddlers are especially prone to constipation and often do not pass a stool for many days. These problems often start around toilet training time. If your child produces stools infrequently, the stools become hard and cause pain when they are passed. Consequently your child may become scared to pass stools and will hold in the stools as long as possible. This only worsens the problem. This often leads to recurrent bouts of abdominal pain. **Treatment of this problem should be discussed with your child's doctor** and should consist of appropriate changes in diet, good toilet habits, and possibly the regular use of stool softeners and laxatives until the problem is resolved. **Constipation tends to be a recurring problem** so be on the lookout for relapses.

C) Constipation in older children

Constipation is very common at all ages. Have you watched TV lately and seen all the advertisements for laxatives?

Children with constipation may develop **soiling** and even appear to have **diarrhea!** The sooner these problems are dealt with, the sooner they will go away! They seldom resolve on their own and you will need expert help and guidelines on the appropriate diet, good toilet habits, and the use of stool softeners and laxatives.

D) Constipation while traveling

Constipation is an extremely common problem when traveling. The excitement and the stresses of travel, changes in diet, and erratic availability of toilet facilities all contribute to a tendency to constipation. Regular toilet habits are extremely important and attention to these as well as an appropriate diet will go a long way in preventing constipation and bouts of abdominal pain. Make sure all the travelers in your party keep up their fluid intake, eat fiber-containing foods, and have regular bathroom breaks. It's a good idea to include a stool softener and laxative in your travel kit.

NOTE:
Although fruit juices are very helpful in the treatment of constipation, they are very poor sources of nutrition for an infant and young growing child. In the long term, fruit juice should not take the place of breast-milk, formula, or ordinary milk in your child's diet.

HEADACHE

Children fairly commonly complain of headaches, and this usually does not indicate a severe underlying disease such as a brain tumor. Many headaches occur in association with other illnesses such as infections, for example strep throat. They may also occur with sinusitis, earache, and other infectious diseases that have nothing to do with the head.

Very young children have trouble localizing pain and may complain of a headache when, in fact, they have abdominal pain.

Headaches are often a manifestation of the psychological stresses of life. The stresses of travel often cause headaches in the entire family!

Recurrent headaches are often due to migraine or tension and these should be discussed with your child's physician. Migraine headaches are often located in the front of the head, often behind an eye. They are frequently throbbing in nature and may be associated with visual symptoms, nausea, and vomiting.

On occasion, there is a serious cause for a headache. If your child complains of a severe headache, has a fever, neck stiffness, or is confused, then immediate medical attention should be sought. Your child is unlikely to have meningitis if she is alert and active and is happily watching TV and interacting with her environment!

Treatment.

Initial treatment of a headache, without other symptoms, should consist of an appropriate dose of acetaminophen or ibuprofen. Ibuprofen tends to be more effective than acetaminophen for migraine headaches. Having your child lie down in a dark room will also often help the headache. Headaches that do not respond to these simple measures should be discussed with your child's physician.

If your child complains of a headache but wants to watch TV or play Nintendo, he does **not** have a significant headache and there may be an ulterior motive for the headache!

CONVULSIONS/SEIZURES

Three to four percent of children have convulsions associated with fevers. (See section on fever, page 211.) These seizures are usually short, lasting only a few minutes, do not cause brain damage and are known as **febrile seizures.**

Some children have **recurrent seizures** unassociated with fever. When a child has recurrent seizures they are said to have epilepsy. This child should be seen by a neurologist and will probably be maintained on appropriate anti-convulsant medication.

Occasionally, a child who has never had seizures before will develop prolonged seizures. Such a child may have a serious disease such as meningitis, a brain hemorrhage, or poisoning and requires immediate medical care.

First aid treatment for a seizure is as follows:

1. Try not to panic.

2. Lie your child down on his side and make sure that his head is lower than the rest of his body so that any mucus or vomit can drain out. Position your child's head so that the head is slightly tilted back. This will help maintain an open airway.

3. Do **not** attempt to force hard objects, such as rulers or pencils, between your child's teeth. Do **not** attempt to give anything by mouth.

4. If your child has a fever, remove your child's clothing. If your child is prone to febrile seizures, insert an acetaminophen suppository if this is available.

5. If the seizure persists for longer than five to ten minutes, then seek immediate medical attention. Call 911.

Remember that most seizures are short and do **not** cause brain damage. There are, however, very important causes for seizures such as meningitis or clots on the brain. Therefore, medical attention should always be sought after your child has had a convulsion. The exception to this is the child with known febrile seizures who, shortly after the seizure, is alert, running around, and does not show any signs of illness. Even then it is preferable to discuss the episode with your child's doctor, as the illness that caused the fever may need to be treated.

If your child has a **recurrent seizure disorder (epilepsy)** and you plan to **travel,** make sure you take sufficient anti-seizure medication with you on your travels. Depending on your child's seizure medication, it may be a good idea to have your child's anti-convulsant blood level checked prior to departure. Have a supply of **rectal diazepam available** to treat any prolonged seizures. You should know how to use the rectal diazepam. Ask your physician about this.

If your child is prone to febrile seizures, at the first sign of an illness such as an upper respiratory infection, keep your child lightly dressed and give your child an appropriate dose of a fever-reducing medication such as acetaminophen (*Tylenol*) or ibuprofen (*Advil* or *Motrin*). If your child has a fever and refuses to take medication by mouth or is confused, insert an acetaminophen suppository. Rectal diazepam may also be useful in the child with recurrent febrile seizures, especially if the seizures tend to be prolonged.

SKIN RASHES

The skin is the largest organ in the body so it is not surprising that a lot can go wrong with it! Skin rashes may be an indication of a skin disease only or they may be just the tip of the iceberg and reflect an underlying, more generalized disease. Many infectious diseases present with a rash and a fever. These may be relatively minor illnesses or very severe illnesses such as dengue fever or meningococcemia, both of which may be acquired while traveling. If your child has a rash and is ill, medical care should be sought.

Discussed below are a few of the more common skin ailments that your child is likely to get. Other skin problems are discussed elsewhere in the book.

Diaper dermatitis.

Most young children get a diaper rash at sometime or another. This is not surprising since diapers are receptacles for urine and feces! Children who don't wear diapers don't get diaper rashes! Young children tend to have very sensitive and delicate skins and diaper rashes can develop very rapidly, often overnight or after just one or two loose stools. Some children get diaper rashes very easily despite good hygiene. Diaper rashes are caused by irritants in the urine or stools and by infectious agents, bacteria, fungi (yeasts), and viruses. Rashes often occur when new foods are introduced into the diet. Acidic foods such as citrus fruits or tomatoes are particularly likely to cause rashes when first introduced. Sometimes rashes are caused by irritation from the diaper itself. If you have recently changed diaper brands and your child develops a diaper rash, it may be prudent to go back to the old brand.

Prevention of diaper rashes

Most diaper rashes can be prevented by good hygiene.

— **Change your child's diaper frequently,** preferably as soon as it is wet or soiled.

— If your child has soiled, **cleanse** the area gently with wet wipes or tap water and a cotton ball. It is not necessary to use soap after every bowel movement. Use soap only if the stool does not come off easily and then use only a mild soap such as *Dove*.

— Allow the diaper area to air frequently. Keep the diaper area uncovered as often and as long as possible. This is often easier said than done! Do not fasten the diaper so that it is airtight, especially overnight.

— **Do not overuse wet wipes,** as these may dry out the skin. Do not use scented wet wipes.

— **Antibiotics and diaper rashes.** If your child is put on an antibiotic, give your child yogurt that contains a live culture. Change the diaper more frequently, especially if your child develops diarrhea. Use a barrier cream such as those mentioned below. If your child develops a diaper rash, consider using an over the counter anti-fungal cream or ointment such as *Lotrimin*. A yeast diaper rash is suggested by a bright red rash which is worse in the creases and has scattered satellite spots around it.

— Do not use plastic waterproof pants over cloth diapers.

— **Barrier creams and ointments** may help to prevent diaper rashes and are useful as part of the treatment of diaper rashes. Most infants do not need to have one of these ointments or creams applied routinely, but just if the skin is becoming irritated. It is often a good idea to apply these preventively overnight. Many of these contain zinc oxide or petro-

latum or both. Some well-known brands are *Desitin,
A & D ointment,* and *Triple Paste,* the last being particularly effective. Probably one of the most effective
barrier agents available is *Bentonite* paste, but you
will need to ask your pharmacist to make this up. You
do not need a prescription for any of these agents.

— Disposable diapers, especially the more absorbent
varieties, are more effective in preventing diaper
rashes than cloth diapers, so consider changing to
these if your child is prone to diaper rashes.

— Get your child out of diapers as soon as possible. Children who don't wear diapers do not get diaper rashes!

Treatment of diaper rashes

— Follow the preventative measures mentioned above.

— Expose the diaper area to the air more frequently.

— If your child's skin is too sensitive to touch, use a
spray bottle of water to clean the skin after soiling.
Fill a spray bottle with ½ tsp baking soda dissolved in
16 oz. warm water. Spray vigorously to remove stool
and urine.

— Allow to air dry or pat dry gently. It is not necessary
to remove all of the barrier cream at every change.

— Use one of the barrier creams described above. For
severe diaper rashes consider using *Triple Paste* or
Bentonite ointment. If the diaper rash persists, try an
antifungal cream such as *Lotrimin.*

— If you have been using cloth diapers, try one of the
newer, more absorbent disposable diapers.

— A weak steroid cream such as ½% or 1% hydrocortisone may help to decrease the inflammation but
should be used **in combination** with other creams

and ointments and **only** after consultation with a physician. Unless directed by a physician, do **not** use potent steroid creams in the diaper area as the steroid may be absorbed into the body and cause serious side effects.

Note: Consult a physician if:

— The rash persists or gets worse.

— There are large blisters in the diaper area.

— Your child appears ill.

Dry Skin and Eczema (Atopic Dermatitis).

Many people have a tendency to develop dry skin. Children are no different and may be even more prone to dry skin and eczema, especially if they have an allergic family history. When skin is dry it tends to itch. Scratching leads to rashes and often to skin infections, the most common being impetigo. Dry skin and eczema often have a genetic basis so they tend to run in families. There are ways you can minimize the discomfort and prevent the skin from drying out:

— When bathing, use a mild soap or a soap-free cleanser such as *Dove Foaming Body Wash* or *Oil of Olay Foaming Body Wash*. Soaps should be free of scents and dyes.

— Wash in warm rather than hot water.

— After bathing or showering, instead of rubbing your child dry with a towel, pat your child dry.

— Apply a moisturizing cream or lotion immediately

after bathing and while your child's skin is still damp. Moisturizing creams tend to be more effective than lotions. Examples of these are *Cetaphil Moisturizing Cream* and *Eucerin Intensive Repair Cream*.

— Reapply these moisturizers liberally and often.

— Wear cool cotton clothes next to the skin. Many people react to wool next to their skin. If the dryness worsens or results in the appearance of circular dry patches or your child scratches excessively, then you should apply an over-the-counter hydrocortisone cream to these dry patches.

— Consider using a humidifier in the bedroom if the air is very dry. Keep the humidity at 35 percent to 40 percent. (If the room humidity is over forty percent the growth of molds and house dust mites will be encouraged and they may increase the risk of asthma and allergies.)

Sometimes a child has more than just dry skin. He may have **eczema.** Eczema in babies often shows up as very dry cheeks, a dry chin and cracked and bleeding areas behind the ears. Later on dry circular patches appear on different parts of the body and may be misdiagnosed as ringworm. In older children, eczema is often worse in the flexures of the elbows and behind the knees. Eczema is much more common in children who come from allergic families and in children who have food allergies or asthma. It is often described as "the itch that rashes." The skin is dry and itchy. Your child scratches and then develops the rash!

If you suspect that your child has eczema you should meet with your child's doctor to draw up an eczema treatment plan. This will usually consist of moisturizing agents, steroid or other anti-inflammatory creams and ointments, and an anti-itch medicine to take by mouth. Effective anti-itch medications include Benadryl and other antihistamines. Eczema may become infected, in which case your doctor may prescribe an antibiotic.

Periodically eczema may flare up and make your child even more unhappy. Causes of such flare-ups include new foods, new detergents, soaps or medications, infections, stress, and allergies. At these times you may need to intensify your child's treatment by applying creams and ointments more frequently, using stronger prescription steroid medications, increasing the dose of the oral anti-itch medications and even trying a course of antibiotics. **Infection** often makes eczema worse and may present as pus-filled blisters, weeping and oozing, or by increased scabbing and crusting.

Hives.

Hives are raised, red and itchy areas which tend to move from one area of the skin to another. There are many causes of hives including allergies (for example to a drug or a food), insect bites or stings and infections. Sometimes physical factors such as changes in temperature or exercise bring out hives. Hives may last for days or weeks and frequently a cause is never found.

Treatment

— Try to identify the trigger and then avoid this. Ask yourself: Is my child on any medication? Has my child eaten a new food? Have I tried a new soap or detergent?

— Give your child an antihistamine such as *Benadryl* or one of the newer non-sedating antihistamines.

— Keep your child as cool as possible. Hot baths or

showers, excessive activity, sleeping in a warm bed at night or being overdressed may all worsen the hives.

— If your child is ill or has a fever that lasts more than three to four days, medical care should be sought.

NOTE: Some people develop hives as part of a more severe, generalized allergic reaction. **If your child's lips swell or if there is any breathing or swallowing difficulty, seek medical attention immediately! If you have an *Epipen* injector, use it immediately!**

Heat rash/prickly heat. See section on traveling and rashes, page 148.

Folliculitis and boils. See section on traveling and rashes, page 149.

Impetigo. See section on traveling and rashes, page 150.

Fungal infections, including ringworm and athletes foot. See section on traveling and rashes, page 152.

Sunburn. See section on sunburn, page 299.

Poison ivy and contact dermatitis. See section on poison ivy, page 324.

Scabies. See section on foreign adoptions, page 189.

Lice/nits. See section on foreign adoptions, page 190.

Insect and tick bites. See sections on insect and tick bites, as well as section on preventing insect and tick bites, page 312.

Foot blisters. See section on foot care, page 350.

4

Summer Woes

SUNBURN/SUN PROTECTION

What is sunburn?

We have probably all been sunburned at one time or another and we know what causes it! Sunburn is due to overexposure to the ultraviolet rays of the sun. Mild sunburn is equivalent to a first degree burn and severe, blistering sunburn is equivalent to a second degree burn.

Why all the fuss about sunburn?

Sunburn is probably the most common summer hazard most of us face. It is also one of the more common travel-related conditions. It is often stated that accidents, especially motor-vehicle accidents, are the commonest cause of travel-related deaths. However, some experts say that death from skin cancer attributed to serious sunburns acquired many years earlier while on vacation is an even more common cause of travel-related death!

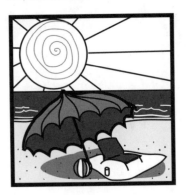

Sun does not only cause **sunburn** but also **aging of the skin** and most importantly, **skin cancer**. The incidence of skin cancer is increasing at a greater rate than that of any other cancer. One in five Americans can expect to develop skin cancer in their lifetime! The most serious type of skin cancer, **melanoma,** is often fatal and may lead to death in early adulthood. The death rate from melanoma has been increasing at a rate of four percent every year since 1973! **Five or more blistering sunburns more than double the risk of getting melanoma later in life.**

It has been estimated that eighty percent of a person's lifetime exposure to the sun has occurred by the age twenty. As a parent, you are in a position to ensure your child's exposure to the sun is limited and safe. **The damage caused by the sun is cumulative and often only shows up years later** with premature aging, wrinkles, sunspots, and cancer. Any tan is a sign of skin damage! Unfortunately, sun damage from sunlight builds up with continued exposure, whether sunburn occurs or not!

Young children are particularly sensitive to the effects of the sun. The skin of infants is thinner and more sensitive than that of adults. The younger the child, the less the protection against the sun and the worse the skin damage. Children also tend to spend more time outdoors than adults. **Sunburn in childhood is more likely to lead to skin cancer than sunburn in adulthood.** The immature eyes of infants are also particularly vulnerable to the effects of the sun's rays.

What is ultraviolet radiation/light?

Ultraviolet light is the light you cannot see and is made up of UVA, UVB, and UVC. UVC is filtered out as it passes through the atmosphere and is not an important factor in sunburn. UVA and UVB have an additive effect on the skin and are responsible for skin damage.

UVB is most responsible for sunburn and the later development of skin cancer and cataracts. UVB is most potent in the middle of the day. UVA is mainly responsible for skin aging (wrinkles, sagging, and brown sun spots), but also plays a part in the development of sunburn and skin cancer. UVA is present throughout the day and penetrates more deeply into the body's subcutaneous tissues. UVA is also harmful to the eyes and contributes to snow blindness and to the formation of cataracts. Unlike UVB, UVA is transmitted through window glass.

Heat, humidity, and wind can increase the effects of ultraviolet radiation. So does reflection of UV rays from snow and water. Moist skin reflects less ultraviolet rays so allows greater absorption of ultraviolet rays.

The UV index: This is often published daily in the newspaper and will give you some idea of the amount of ultraviolet radiation that day. The scale is from 1 to 10. The higher the number, the greater the risk.

Prevention of sunburn.

As with all accidents and illnesses, prevention is the best medicine. **Avoiding sun damage should involve a *total* program, not just the use of sunscreens!**

1. Limit exposure to the sun.

- **Minimize the amount of time spent in the sun.** This is especially important early on in the season when the skin is particularly sensitive. Increase sun exposure by a few minutes each day.

- **Avoid deliberate sunbathing.**

- **Stay out of the sun at the hottest times of the day.** UVB is most severe in the middle of the day (10 AM–4 PM). "Only mad dogs and Englishmen go out in the noonday sun." A good rule of thumb is that if your shadow is shorter than you are, you should not be out in the sun. Plan your outdoor activities for early or late in the day.

- It is important to remember that **you can still get severely sunburned on cloudy days,** as seventy to eighty percent of the UVB can get through the clouds. Remember, ultraviolet rays are invisible and can be reflected from the surfaces around you.

- **The higher the altitude, the more severe the effects of the sun.**

    Sun exposure increases by at least four percent for each 1,000 foot of elevation. In other words, at an altitude of 10,000 feet your body is exposed to forty percent more UVB than it is at sea level. At higher altitudes and during the winter there is less atmospheric ozone to protect you. You may get as much UVB exposure in snowy Vail, Colorado (altitude 8,500 feet) as you would get on a sunny day in Orlando, Florida! Skiers and mountain climbers are particularly prone to sunburn, not only because of the high altitude, but also because of the reflected rays from the snow.

- You don't have to be in direct sunlight to get sunburned. **Sun may be reflected** from concrete, water, snow, or sand and burn you even though you wear a hat or are beneath a beach umbrella.

2. Clothing and hats.

- **Wearing protective clothing is an essential part of sun protection.**

- Not all clothing offers equal protection against the sun. Your child could still get sunburned through clothing! A thin, white cotton T-shirt has only an SPF (sun protection factor) of 5. If clothing becomes wet, the SPF is decreased. **The tighter the weave and the darker the color, the greater the protection against UV rays.** Before you buy, hold the garment up to a light source. If little light gets through, you have made a good choice. You can purchase light-weight, sun-protective clothing from *Sun Precautions (Solumbra clothing*—(800) 882-7860). Sun-protective clothes have a label listing the garment's UV protection factor (UPF) value. **Blue denim has a very high UPF value.**

- Long-sleeved shirts and long pants will give added protection.

- Clothing that is loose-fitting is generally cooler and offers better protection against the sun than does tight-fitting clothing.

- Your child should wear a **wide-brimmed hat** with a brim of at least three inches. Baseball caps give very little sun protection to the face if worn backwards!

3. Use a sunscreen or a sunblock.

- There are two main types of sunscreen. They include:

    Chemical sunscreens. These absorb UV radiation before it penetrates your skin. They tend to be light and easy to apply but **must be applied at least thirty minutes prior to sun exposure.**

    Chemical sunscreens contain a variety of chemicals to block UVB. Some contain chemicals such as Avobenzone (Parsol 1789) to block UVA as well.

Physical sunblocks. These are opaque and physically block, reflect, and scatter the sun's rays.

Physical sunscreens usually contain titanium dioxide and/or zinc oxide. They tend to be messy and uncomfortable, although newer micronized sunblocks which have very fine particles of titanium dioxide or zinc oxide are more user-friendly.

Sunblocks are especially useful on areas such as the nose, cheeks, lips, and tops of the ears and in people allergic to chemical sunscreens. They give immediate protection and do not have to be applied thirty minutes before sun exposure. Sunblocks block UVB and UVA.

- **Always buy a sunscreen that blocks both UVA and UVB.** Most sunscreens are more effective in blocking UVB than UVA. (The SPF rating only applies to UVB.)

- **Use a sunscreen with an SPF of at least 15.** In very sensitive individuals (infants, fair people with blonde or red hair, or people with many freckles or moles), use a sunscreen with an SPF of at least 30.

A sunscreen with an SPF of 15 filters out ninety-three percent of UVB rays **if applied correctly.** A sunscreen with an SPF of 30 filters out ninety-seven percent of UVB rays **if applied correctly.**

Sunscreens with SPFs greater than 30 are probably not necessary and are more expensive. **It is better to buy a larger bottle of sunscreen with a lower SPF and apply it more liberally than to use a sunscreen with a higher SPF and not apply enough!**

The SPF number gives you some idea of how long you can remain in the sun before burning. If, for example, you would normally burn in ten minutes, applying a **sufficient amount** of sunscreen with an SPF of 15 would provide you with about 150 minutes in the sun before burning. **However, most people do not apply enough sunscreen to achieve the labeled SPF!**

The SPF can be reduced by perspiration and swimming.

A sunscreen is said to be *water resistant* if it lasts for forty minutes in water and *waterproof* if it lasts eighty minutes or longer.

- **Apply the sunscreen thirty minutes before being exposed to the sun** to allow time for the lotion to penetrate the skin. In particularly sun-sensitive individuals, reapply the sunscreen just before exposure.

- **Apply sufficient sunscreen.** Most people use ¼ to ½ the recommended amount of sunscreen. An adult needs at least 1 oz. (1 palmful) of lotion to cover the body completely. If the sunscreen is applied at least twice a day, an eight ounce bottle of lotion would be expected to last only four days!

- **Cover all parts of the body exposed to the sun.** Apply an especially thick layer to the shoulders and to the nose. **Do not forget the tips of the ears, the neck, ankles, and the tops of the feet.** Apply a sunblock or lip balm with sunscreen to the lips.

- **Reapply the sunscreen frequently,** at least every two hours. Reapply more frequently if sweating excessively or swimming. Reapply after toweling or when clothing rubs off the sunscreen, for example, when hiking. Waterproof sunscreens will last longer in water but even then need to be reapplied frequently.

- Sunscreens may cause allergic or irritant rashes. Sunscreens containing PABA have a greater chance of causing allergic rashes. To avoid this, choose a sunscreen that contains PABA esters or other ingredients. You can do a **patch test** by applying a small amount to the inside of the forearm first and noting any redness or irritation.

- **Sunscreen does NOT allow unlimited sun exposure.** It merely helps to decrease sunburn. If you would normally get sunburned in ten minutes and you have applied a **sufficient amount** of sunscreen with an SPF of 15, you **may** be able to spend 150 minutes in the sun. Once you have spent your 150 minutes in the sun you need to cover up or get out of the sun. Reapplying the sunscreen does **not** allow you to spend another 150 minutes in the sun!

   In other words, sunscreen should *not* be used to prolong time spent in the sun.

We should all try to adopt the Australian slogan, **"Slip on a shirt, slop on sunscreen, and slap on a hat!"** (Slip, slop, slap!)

Special situations.

1. **Infants.** Infants are especially prone to severe sunburn. Many sunscreen bottles state "not for use below 6 months of age." Most sunscreens can be used on infants and it is far better to use a sunscreen than let your infant get sunburned. It is better still **not** to expose young infants to the sun, especially in the middle of the day. If you have no option, use a sunscreen as well as clothing that covers the arms and legs. Shield your child with an umbrella and use a head covering as well.
2. **Adolescents.** Adolescents are especially fond of getting suntans. I don't know of any way to convince teenagers of

the dangers of the sun, but do try to teach them how to limit sun exposure and how to use sunscreen correctly.

3. **Indoor tanning devices and tanning salons can be as harmful as direct sunlight!** Most tanning salons use lamps that supposedly only emit UVA rays, but many lamps are not well calibrated and emit UVB rays as well.

4. **Sunscreen and insect repellants.** It is preferable not to use lotions that contain both a sunscreen and an insect repellant. You should use each separately. **Apply the sunscreen first** and allow time for it to penetrate the skin. Apply the insect repellant over the sunscreen just before exposure. Do not rub the repellent into the skin. **The repellent will reduce the SPF of the sunscreen.**

5. **Medications and sun sensitivity.** Some medications increase sensitivity to the sun. This is especially true of some antibiotics but also anti-inflammatories, oral contraceptives, and some diuretics.

6. **Dark skinned people.** It is a fallacy that dark skinned races can't get sunburned or get skin cancer. They should also follow safe sun rules.

How to _treat_ sunburn.

Unfortunately, the symptoms of sunburn do not begin until two to four hours after the sun's damage has already been done. The peak reaction of redness, pain, and swelling does not occur for twenty-four hours. In other words, you will not realize your child has been sunburned until after the fact. **Nothing can reverse the effects of sunburn that has already occurred.** The damage is done! You can, however, treat the symptoms. The following measures may help:

• Cool baths or wet compresses are very effective in relieving pain and burning.

- Ibuprofen or acetaminophen may help relieve the sensation of pain and heat.

- Non-prescription 1% hydrocortisone cream and bland moisturizing creams can be applied two to three times a day and may help to decrease pain and swelling. Refrigerating creams and lotions prior to use gives added relief. Aloe vera gel or cream is soothing and may aid healing.

- Get your child to drink extra fluid to prevent dehydration.

- Peeling of the skin may occur some days after sunburn. The itching can be partly relieved by applying moisturizing creams and lotions frequently.

    > A variety of other topical remedies are often recommended. These include oatmeal or baking soda baths, aloe vera, vitamin E oil, and many other creams and lotions. Remember, the skin has already been damaged and can easily be further irritated! Probably very little else is as soothing as cool water soaks and compresses. Some physicians recommend high-dose ibuprofen or oral corticosteroids but there is little scientific evidence to substantiate that they are effective once the sunburn has already occurred. They also may have unpleasant side effects!

NOTES:

- Do **not** apply ointments, petroleum products, or butters to sunburn because they all prevent heat and sweat from escaping from the skin.

- Do **not** use first aid creams or sprays that contain benzocaine because they may cause allergic rashes.

- **Do not apply DEET-containing insect repellents to sunburned skin.** Damaged skin allows greater absorption of substances into the body.
- If your child has blisters, do **not** pop them. Once they are broken, cut away the dead skin and try to discourage your child from picking at the peeling edges until the skin has healed completely. Some physicians recommend applying a topical antibiotic such as *Bacitracin* to the exposed new skin, but this is seldom necessary as secondary infection is uncommon.

The most important aspect of the treatment is preventing further sun damage! Do *not* expose your child to the sun again until the skin is completely healed.

WHEN TO SEEK MEDICAL ATTENTION

1. If your child has extensive blistering.
2. If your child appears ill or dizzy. A severe sunburn may be as serious as a severe burn from a hot liquid or other heat sources and may lead to fluid loss and shock.
3. If your child has a temperature over 102 degrees Fahrenheit.
4. If the sunburn appears to have become infected. Fortunately this is rare.

IN SUMMARY

- Exposure to too much sunlight is dangerous to your child's health, both in the short-term and the long-term. The good news is that minimizing ultraviolet radiation during the first twenty years of life will decrease your child's risk of developing skin cancer and melanoma later on. Using the common sense precautions suggested above, will help prevent sun damage.

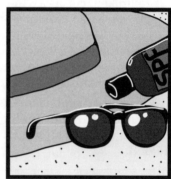

- **Sunscreens alone will *not* provide sufficient protection.**

- Children raised in households where putting on sunscreen is as routine as brushing teeth will find it easier to continue the habit even into adolescence. If **you** set a good example for your children when they are young, they are more likely to continue these habits into adolescence and adulthood.

- **There is no such thing as a healthy tan!**

Sunlight-related eye diseases/sunglasses.

Just as the sun's rays may cause damage to the skin, they may also cause damage to the eyes, increasing the chance that your child will develop **cataracts** later in life. Chronic sun exposure also increases the risk of macular degeneration which is a significant cause of blindness in the elderly. The **acute effects** of the sun on the eye are **photoconjunctivitis** (inflammation of the conjunctiva) and **photokeratitis** (inflammation of the cornea). These are the equivalent of sunburn of the eye. The eyes will be red and very painful but these conditions do **not** usually lead to long-term eye damage. **Snow blindness** is a very severe form of photokeratitis.

Choosing sunglasses

— Buy sunglasses with lenses that absorb ninety-nine to a hundred percent of UV radiation. Look for labels that say "photo, UV absorption up to 400 nm," "maximum or 99% UV protection or blockage," "special purpose," or "meets ANSI (American National Standard Institute) UV requirements."

— The larger the lenses and the closer they are to the eye, the better the protection.

— The darkness of the lenses does **not** correlate with the ability to block UV rays.

Cheap toy sunglasses should be avoided. They give little or no protection and may harm your child's eyes further by encouraging him to look into the sun.

PROTECTING YOUR CHILD AGAINST INSECT BITES, TICK BITES, AND INSECT STINGS

See also: Section on malaria. (page 142)
Section on Lyme disease. (page 342
Section on West Nile fever. (page 339)

The pleasures of the outdoors are often spoiled by the unwelcome attention of biting and stinging insects. Fortunately, in the United States, most bites and stings are harmless and cause only minor local irritation. In contrast, in many other parts of the world, diseases transmitted by insects are a major health hazard and cause severe illness and chronic ill health as well as millions of deaths. It is important to remember, however, that even in the United States insects and ticks may carry serious diseases. Mosquitoes may cause West Nile fever and ticks may cause Lyme disease, Rocky Mountain spotted fever and a number of other illnesses.

Stinging insects usually just inflict unpleasant and painful stings which get your attention immediately. A small number of people, however, have severe reactions to bee stings which may be life-threatening. Others, especially children, have fairly significant local allergic skin reactions to bites from common insects such as gnats, mosquitoes, or fleas. Insect stings tend to cause immediate and noticeable pain; on the other hand, insect and tick bites are usually painless and at first go unnoticed. Even spider bites may not cause much pain initially but severe local pain, redness, and swelling may develop later along with more general symptoms such as headache, abdominal pain, and muscle cramps.

The measures you and your child need to take to prevent insect and tick bites depend largely on the diseases you are trying to prevent. It is extremely important to take preventative measures seriously if you are in an area where you might acquire serious diseases such as malaria or yellow fever. Malaria causes three million deaths each year!

Just as the prevention of sunburn involves more than just one application of sunscreen, so the prevention of insect bites and stings involves more than just the use of repellents.

A) General measures to minimize the chance of insect and tick bites and stings.

1. **Choose your picnic/camp site carefully.** Avoid places that attract insects such as fields of clover, orchards with fallen fruit, and areas near trash cans. Also avoid areas with dense vegetation. High and dry areas that have less vegetation are less likely to harbor insects and ticks. Breezes may deter flying insects.

2. When camping, do not sleep or lie right on the ground but rather on a blanket or camping mattress.

3. Avoid bright clothing and jewelry, perfumes, aftershave lotions, hair spray, scented cosmetics, and soaps, all of which tend to attract insects.

4. **Dress sensibly.** Wear closed shoes, long-sleeved shirts, and long pants. Tuck the bottom of pants into socks or boots. Loose fitting clothes are better as mosquitoes may bite right through tight fitting clothing. Insects tend to be attracted more to dark-colored clothing than light-colored clothing. It is

also easier to spot ticks and other insects on light-colored clothing. Good colors are khaki, tan, and white. Wearing a **hat,** especially with permethrin sprayed on it will help greatly in preventing insect "attacks" on your head.

5. When eating outside in the company of bees and other insects, eat and drink cautiously. Cover food and drinks and be careful when drinking directly from soda pop cans. Bees, especially yellow jackets, often crawl inside open cans to feed.

6. Avoid rapid movements when in areas with many bees. If a bee lands on your child, do not slap or brush it away. Bees don't usually sting unless frightened or provoked.

7. Keep insects out of your car. Travel with your windows closed. Keep a cloth or towel handy to trap bees or other flying insects. Pull off the road before attempting to get rid of an intruder.

8. Some insects, especially mosquitoes, only feed at certain times. The mosquito that carries malaria usually feeds between dusk and dawn, so try not to be outdoors at these times. The mosquito that transmits West Nile fever is most active in the early morning and at dusk.

9. In your own backyard, get rid of standing water, where insects can breed.

10. If in tick-infested areas, perform careful body inspections twice a day for ticks.

B) Insect repellents and insecticides.

Insect repellents are usually applied directly to the skin and repel insects and ticks. Insecticides are usually applied to clothing or sprayed into confined spaces and often kill insects or ticks. The repellent you choose will vary according to a number of factors:

- The **"bug"** you are trying to repel and the **illness** you are trying to prevent.
- **How long** you need the repellent to be effective.
- **Your location.** For example, you will need a more potent repellent in a rain forest where the concentration of "bugs" is high and where rain and sweat will tend to wash the repellent away.
- The **age** of the person using it. The younger the child, the more important it is to avoid repellents with high concentrations of DEET.
- **Generally speaking, if it is important to prevent being bitten, you cannot beat the combination of DEET on the skin and permethrin on clothes.**

The time of day that the repellant is applied will vary according to the disease you are trying to avoid. For example, when trying to avoid malaria, the repellant should be applied between dusk and dawn. On the other hand, if you are trying to avoid being bitten by the mosquito which causes yellow fever or dengue fever, you will need to have repellant on during daylight hours as well.

TYPES OF INSECT REPELLANTS AND INSECTICIDES

1. DEET

There are many types of insect repellants, but the most reliable and effective **by far** are those that contain DEET (N, N-diethyl-3-methylbenzamide). However, these may be toxic to young children if not used correctly, as DEET is absorbed through the skin into the circulatory system.

It is generally safer for children to use preparations that contain less than 30% DEET. The main drawback of using preparations that contain less than 30% DEET is that they do not last as long as the repellents with higher concentrations and therefore need to be reapplied more often.

DEET preparations are available in many forms including sticks, sprays, creams and lotions. The concentration of DEET in these preparations range from 5% to 100%. The duration of action generally correlates with the concentration up to 50%. There is not much point in using preparations with concentrations in excess of 50%. Some of the lotions are available as **extended-release formulations:**

- **Ultrathon.** This is one of the more effective preparations and is an excellent choice, especially in adolescents and adults and when it is vital to prevent insect bites. This contains 33% DEET and can be purchased through Travel Medicine [(800) 872-8633, and http:// www.travmed.com]. It is used by the military and is extremely effective, providing up to twelve hours of protection (the same as preparations containing 75% DEET).

- Another very effective and long-lasting preparation of DEET for use on both children and adults is *Sawyer-controlled release insect repellant* **(20% DEET)** [(800) 940-4464, www.sawyeronline.com]. This lotion is easy to apply and **minimizes the absorption of DEET.** It lasts up to five hours and is probably the best choice for children.

    The American Academy of Pediatrics recommends using preparations that contain less than 30% DEET. It also states that DEET should not be used in children younger than two months of age.

To be effective, repellants **must be applied to all exposed skin,** as mosquitoes will readily bite unprotected skin just and inch or two away from the treated area. Ideally, especially in children, DEET should only be applied once a day to limit its potential toxicity. However, preparations with lower concentrations of DEET may need to be reapplied more often, particularly if your child is sweating or very active.

NOTES:

- Avoid applying DEET around the eyes or mouth.
- Do not apply DEET to the hands of small children as they often put their hands and fingers in their mouths.
- Do not apply to cuts, wounds, sunburned or irritated skin.
- When applying DEET, do **not** rub it in but apply it lightly.
- Do not let young children apply DEET themselves.
- Only apply DEET to exposed skin and not under clothing.
- Do not reapply DEET unless necessary.
- Do not spray DEET near food.
- **Wash off the repellant with soap and water when it is no longer needed.**
- Keep DEET-containing products in a safe place where young children cannot reach of them.

DEET is combustible and is **highly toxic if ingested,** so keep it in a safe place away from the inquisitive hands of children.

DEET can also be applied to clothing, although it may damage plastics and spandex. It may also damage wrist watch crystals and eyeglass frames. It is generally preferable to use DEET on skin and permethrin on clothing. DEET does not damage natural fibers such as wool or cotton.

Overall, DEET is extremely safe in children if used correctly. It is the best preparation to use when trying to prevent bites from insects that carry dangerous diseases such as malaria.

2. Other repellents

Many other insect repellents are available, some of which contain only "natural" substances. These include citronella, which is found in Avon's *Skin So Soft*. A testament to the fact that this preparation is not very effective is that Avon has recently introduced a new formulation of *Skin So Soft* that contains DEET. One of the more effective "green" formulations is ***Bite Blocker*** which contains soybean oil, geranium oil, and coconut oil (http://www.biteblocker.com). Use this preparation if you feel you cannot use a DEET-containing preparation. If you use these products it is important to **reapply** them **frequently** because of their short duration of action. In some cases, for example, if you use citronella, you will need to apply the preparation hourly. However, none of these natural preparations is as effective or lasts as long as DEET which remains the "gold standard."

> New insect repellents on the horizon contain picardin (*Bayrepel, Autan Repel*) and may turn out to be as effective as DEET.

3. Insecticides: permethrin-containing products

Permethrin is extremely effective in protecting against ticks and also against many biting insects, including mosquitoes. In fact, it is more effective against ticks than DEET. It should **not** be applied directly to the skin but should be applied to clothing, bedding, bed nets, and camping gear. It does **not** damage fabrics and will last through many washes. In areas with a high concentration of ticks and Lyme disease, spray permethrin on socks, shoes, and trousers, and even consider ankle bands saturated with permethrin. When spraying clothes, hold the can about twelve inches away and use enough spray to moisten the entire garment. Spray both sides and let the clothing dry before wearing.

It is especially important to spray permethrin on bed nets when trying to prevent being bitten by the anopheles mosquito which carries malaria. Recommended permithrin-containing preparations to use on clothes and camping equipment include *Sawyer Permethrin Tick Repellent* (800) 356-7811, http://www.sawyeronline.com), *Duranon, Cutter Outdoorsman Gear Guard,* and *Fite Bite Permethrin Solution* (800) TRAV-MED).

Aerosol knock-down insecticides frequently contain permithrin-related substances. Examples of these include *Doom* and *Raid,* which are effective and can be sprayed in the bedroom before going to bed.

An ideal combination for preventing bites of insect and ticks is to use DEET on the skin and permethrin on clothing.

NOTE

Neither DEET nor permethrin protect against stinging insects such as bees, wasps, hornets, or fire ants.

---

4. Folk remedies

Vitamin B1 and garlic by mouth are **NOT** effective repellents. The latter may have repellent effects on the human species! Sucking on lemons may prevent scurvy but not insect bites!

Simultaneous use of sunscreens and insect repellants.

If your child requires both a sunscreen and an insect repellant, it is preferable to use each separately. Apply the sunscreen to your child's skin about thirty minutes prior to sun exposure, allowing time for it to be absorbed by the skin. Then apply the insect repellant. However, the DEET will lessen the protective effects of the sunscreen so it may be advisable to use a sunscreen with a higher SPF than you usually use. An alternative but less ideal approach is to use combination products that contain both DEET and a sunscreen with a SPF of 15 or greater. Examples of such preparations are: *OFF! Skintastic with Sunscreen* (SPF 30) and *Cutter with Sunscreen*. You will need to be cautious about reapplying these preparations to avoid DEET toxicity.

In summary, it is better to use a combination of methods to prevent insect and tick bites and the diseases they transmit.

- Avoid infested habitats.
- Wear suitable clothing.
- Use an effective repellent.
- Apply an insecticide to your clothing, bedding, bed nets, and so on.

Remember, if you are not bitten by the "bug," you won't get the disease!

If you develop any unusual symptoms such as high fevers, severe headache, unusual rashes, etc. after being in an infested area, seek medical attention. Be sure to tell your doctor about your travels.

Never underestimate biting and stinging "critters."

TICK BITES AND TICK REMOVAL

See: Section on prevention of insect and tick bites.
(page 321)
Section on Lyme disease. (page 342)

Tick bites and tick-borne illnesses are common throughout the world, including the United States. In fact, ticks cause almost as many human diseases worldwide as mosquitoes do. In the United States ticks are responsible for more disease than mosquitoes. Ticks transmit a variety of infectious illnesses, with Lyme disease being by far the most common. Another important tick-borne disease in the United States is Rocky Mountain spotted fever.

Prevention of tick bites.

The most important measures here are:
- If possible, avoid tick-infested areas. Be especially vigilant when walking in long grass. Ticks do not jump, or fly, or drop from trees. Ticks crawl on to you as you lie on the ground or stride through long grass, or brush against vegetation.
- Wear suitable clothing and enclosed shoes. Wear long pants and tuck them into socks or boots.
- Apply **permithrin** to clothing.
- Apply a repellent to exposed skin.
- Do twice-daily tick inspections. Remember, the tick stage that usually transmits Lyme disease is the nymph, which is very small—about the size of a sesame seed.

What to do if you find a tick.

If you detect the tick early, it may not be attached and you may be able to pick it off very easily. If the tick is firmly attached, you will need to use tweezers or one of the instruments specifically designed to remove ticks. If using tweezers, grasp the tick as close to your skin as possible and pull upwards and back-

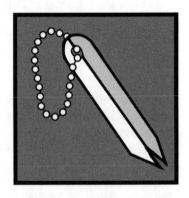

wards with steady, even traction. Do not twist, jerk, squeeze, crush, or puncture the tick. You can purchase instruments specifically designed to remove ticks (Pro-Tick Remedy (800) PIX-TICK/(800) 749-8425, http://www.tickinfo.com). These instruments are particularly useful for removing very small ticks and also lessen the chances of crushing the tick. Once the tick has been removed, disinfect the area with soap and water or an alcohol swab. You may also apply an antibacterial cream such as *triple antibiotic* or *Neosporin.* Discourage your child from scratching the area as this may lead to secondary infection. Occasionally the head of the tick may be left behind in the skin. It is not usually worth the extra trauma of digging it out. Apply an anti-bacterial cream for a few days and the area will usually settle down and clear. Your child may develop a small, red inflamed area or nodule which will disappear over a week or two. This is **not** the rash of Lyme disease.

NOTES:

- If the typical rash of Lyme disease develops in the ensuing days or weeks seek medical attention. Also seek medical attention if your child becomes ill. Refer to the section on Lyme disease for further details, page 342.

- **By far the majority of tick bites in the United States are harmless and do not lead to any disease.** At the most your child will develop a small red area, smaller than a nickel.

- **Deer ticks need to be attached for at least 24 hours before they can transmit Lyme disease.**

- Except in certain high risk areas most deer ticks do **not** carry Lyme disease.

INSECT STINGS

See also: Section on the prevention of insect bites and insect stings, page 324.

As mentioned before, insect repellents do **not** protect against stinging insects, only against biting insects.

What to do if your child is stung.

- If the insect left a stinger in the skin, remove it immediately. The sooner the stinger is removed the less time the poison has to be injected. Scrape the stinger off with a knife or credit card or fingernail. Avoid squeezing the stinger as this will inject more poison. Yellow jackets and wasps do not leave a stinger and may sting repeatedly.
- Apply ice or a cold pack to the sting site. Cortisone cream will help soothe the sting and decrease itching.
- Diphenhydramine (*Benadryl*) by mouth will decrease the allergic reaction and itching. Newer non-sedating antihistamines should be just as effective and do not need to be given as often.
- Give acetaminophen or ibuprofen for pain.

Signs of a severe allergic reaction include:

- Difficulty swallowing, thick tongue, hoarseness.
- Chest tightness, wheezing, difficulty breathing.
- Confusion, fainting, and collapse.

CALL 911 if your child has any of these symptoms. If you have an Epinephrine kit, use it immediately.

NOTES:

- A child who has had a severe reaction should be seen by a physician who can decide whether the child should receive allergy injections.

- **If your child has had a previous severe generalized reaction, you should ALWAYS carry an emergency epinephrine kit (such as Epipen/Epipen Junior) wherever you go.** This is especially important on trips outdoors, vacations, etc. **Learn how to use this kit.**

Most children will not have a severe reaction but may have an itchy, red swelling which could persist for five to seven days. This swelling may extend far beyond the original sting and be tender, warm, and red. This is known as a large local reaction and does **not** usually indicate that the bite is infected. Continued use of cool compresses and appropriate doses of *Benadryl* or other antihistamines will help. Occasionally, with persistent scratching, children may develop a secondary infection at the site of the sting and may require an antibiotic cream or antibiotics by mouth.

SPIDER BITES

There are over 20,000 species of spiders in the United States and 34,000 worldwide! Many species produce venom **but few species are harmful to humans** either because the fangs are not strong enough to penetrate skin or the venom is not toxic enough. In the United States, however, the black widow spider and the brown recluse spider can cause serious reactions or even death, especially in children. Fortunately, bites by these two spiders are relatively rare and often do not produce serious illness. Though fatalities from spider bites are extremely rare, arachnophobia (fear of spiders) is not!

Spider bites are far less common than insect bites or stings. Rarely is the bite witnessed and so diagnosis is often difficult. Spider bites often occur on parts of the body where clothing is constrictive such as at the sites of cuffs, collars, waistbands, groin etc.

What to do if you suspect your child has been bitten by a venomous spider.

1. If you suspect your child has been bitten by a venomous spider, seek medical attention promptly. **Spider bites may not cause much initial pain and may go unnoticed for some time.**

2. **Local treatment** consists of cleaning the wound, immobilizing the affected limb, and **applying ice.**

3. Administer a pain-relieving medicine such as acetaminophen (*Tylenol*) or ibuprofen (*Advil, Motrin*).

4. Keep your child still to minimize the spread of venom.

5. Your child may need a tetanus shot or tetanus booster.

6. Occasionally, antibiotics may be indicated.

Young children suspected of having been bitten by a black widow spider or a brown recluse spider should be hospitalized for observation and treatment.

Black widow spiders

With its legs extended, the black widow spider is usually about the **size of a quarter.** It is usually shiny black in color and has a red, orange or yellow **hour-glass shaped marking on the underside of the abdomen.** It may be found indoors or outdoors. **Immediate effects** of a black widow bite may be a pin prick or pinch sensation, or the bite may go totally unnoticed. **Usually within an hour or so,** a dull burning or aching pain develops at the site of the bite. This pain may last for days. Redness, itching, and swelling

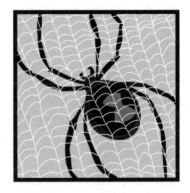

develop and two red **puncture marks may be visible.** These puncture marks are **not** usually visible at the time of the bite. In some people, other more **generalized symptoms** develop later. These symptoms include muscle tremors and aches, cramps, flushing, excessive sweating, and salivation. Swelling of the face, rather like that seen with an allergic reaction, may occur. There may also be chest tightness, backache, **severe abdominal pain,** and fainting. Even more severe symptoms may develop later. By this stage, the victim is hopefully in a hospital. Infants may show none of the above symptoms but just cry inconsolably.

The brown recluse spider

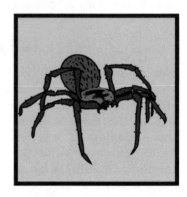

These spiders are smaller than the black widow spiders. With their legs extended they are usually about a size between a nickel and a quarter. They are usually light or dark brown in color and have a violin-shaped mark on their back. They live both indoors and outdoors. They hibernate in the winter so the most likely time for a bite from a brown recluse spider is between April and October. They are more active at night.

Again, the bite may hurt only a little or not at all. Over the next few hours, redness, swelling, and itching may develop, followed by blistering. Two tiny bite marks may be visible. The wound may have the appearance of a **halo** with a blue center surrounded by a white ring which in turn is surrounded by a red ring. The wound often develops a **thick scab (eschar)** which may last for weeks or even longer. When the scab falls off a deep ulcer may be left which may take months to heal. There is usually no immediate danger from a bite from a brown recluse spider as generalized symptoms are rare. However, generalized symptoms may occur in children, especially young children and include fever, nausea, sweating, vomiting and muscle spasms.

Other spiders that may cause symptoms in humans include the **Hobo spider** and **Funnel-web** spiders. The symptoms are more local (pain and blistering at the bite site) and generalized symptoms rarely occur.

IN SUMMARY

- If you or your child is bitten by a spider, you will probably not witness the bite.

- Most spider bites are **not** dangerous and just require local treatment in the form of cleansing, ice, and possibly pain medication such as ibuprofen or acetaminophen. Anti-itch medication such as *Benadryl* may also be useful.

- If you suspect your child has been bitten by a black widow or a brown recluse spider, seek medical attention immediately. If there is any doubt, it is still wise to seek medical attention. Muscle aches or weakness, abdominal pain, excessive sweating, or salivation indicate a serious reaction.

- If you have captured the spider it is helpful to take it along with you to the medical professional for identification. When trying to catch the spider, it is important to avoid being bitten yourself!

SNAKE BITES

Most snakes are **not** aggressive and will **not** bite unless disturbed or challenged. Despite all the horrific stories you hear, there are **very few deaths from snake bites in the United States!** There are approximately 45,000 snake bites a year in the United States and only about ten deaths. Mexico has more poisonous species than the United States and up to 150 people die each year from snake bites. Africa has numerous species of snakes, but most are not poisonous. However, you should respect and avoid snakes as some are extremely poisonous. A bite may lead to severe local tissue damage as well as collapse, cardiac arrest, and death.

Remember, as always, **prevention is better than cure.**

- If you are planning a hiking or camping trip, learn beforehand about the type of snakes you are likely to encounter. Knowledge is power: there may not be any poisonous snakes in the area you plan to visit! If you have learned to recognize the poisonous species, and you get bitten by one of them, you will know you need to get to medical care as soon as possible.
- Avoid areas that are known to be snake infested.
- Protect your feet and legs—wear closed shoes or boots and long pants. Tuck your pants into your socks or boots.
- Look where you put your feet and hands! The vine you are you are about to grab onto may not be a vine!
- Be especially careful when disturbing rocks or piles of stones.
- If collecting firewood when it is dark, take a flashlight with you. Always use a flashlight when moving around your campsite at night.
- When camping outdoors, shake out bedding or sleeping bags before going to bed at night.
- Check shoes and boots before putting them on.

- If you come upon a snake, do not disturb it: many snake bites occur when people (usually adolescent or young adult males) "mess around" with snakes.

The medically important species of snakes in North America fall into two families: the **pit vipers** (rattlesnakes, copperheads, cottonmouth water moccasins, and cantils) and the **elapids** (the coral snakes). Rattlesnakes are found in most states in the United States, whereas the coral snakes are more likely to be found in Arizona, the southeastern United States, and Texas. The coral snake is extremely colorful and has red, yellow, and black bands encircling its body. The red and yellow bands touch each other. Some other harmless species of snake also have red, yellow, and black bands, with the red and yellow bands being separated by a black band. **Red on yellow, kill a fellow; red on black, venom lack.**

Venom from pit vipers tends to cause immediate, severe pain followed by discoloration and swelling at the site of the bite. Other symptoms and signs such as nausea and vomiting, weakness, and a metallic taste in the mouth may follow later. On the other hand, the bite of a coral snake may cause minimal pain and swelling at first but many hours later (sometimes as late as twelve hours), the victim may have nausea and vomiting, headache, sweating, pallor, abdominal pain, and difficulty breathing.

Not all snake bites lead to injection of venom. These bites are known as **dry** bites. Coral snakes only effectively envenom forty percent of the time.

What to do if someone in your party is bitten.

- Try to stay calm. Reassure the victim. Remember most snake bites are not poisonous.

- Keep as quiet and as still as possible.
- Keep the affected limb below the level of the heart to minimize absorption of the venom.
- Immobilize the area with a splint. A very effective technique is known as "pressure immobilization." This involves wrapping the entire extremity with an elastic bandage, starting at the bite site and working toward the heart. The entire extremity is then immobilized in a splint.
- **DO NO HARM!** Do **not** incise and try to suck out the poison. Do **not** apply a tight tourniquet.
- If possible, carry the victim out. If this is not possible, walk the victim out slowly.
- Do **NOT** try to catch the snake. Dead snakes may bite reflexively for up to one hour after being killed!
- Seek medical care.

One expert has said that if you have been bitten by a really poisonous snake, the best first aid equipment to have is a set of car keys. In other words, you will need sophisticated medical care which will only be available in a hospital.

INSECT IN THE EAR

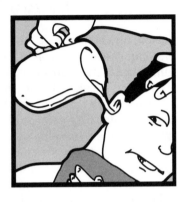

Occasionally while camping or being outdoors, an insect may fly or crawl into your child's ear. This is extremely distressing to the child (as it would be to anyone)! Treatment consists of reassuring your child and gently pouring lukewarm water into the affected ear. The insect will often float out. If the insect does not come out, then medical attention should be sought. Mineral oil can also be poured into the ear in the same fashion to drown the insect. It will then need to be removed by a physician.

Children often put other objects into the ear, favorites being beads and popcorn kernels! Do not attempt to get these foreign bodies out; seek medical attention. Do **not** put sharp objects into the ear or try to remove the foreign body with a paper clip or similar "instrument"!

POISON IVY/CONTACT DERMATITIS

Poison ivy, poison oak, and sumac all have sap (resins) that can cause severe skin rashes. These plants are found throughout the continental United States but not in Hawaii or Alaska. These three plants cause by far the majority of allergic skin rashes due to plants in the United States. About fifty percent of the adult population is sensitive to the resin (uroshiol) found in these plants. The intact plant does not cause rashes but when the plant is damaged, the sap leaks out and if it comes into contact with the skin causes the severe skin rash that follows. Contact with a damaged stem or root will have a similar effect.

A person may also come into contact with the sap on pets, articles of clothing, or tools. Smoke from burning plants is another way in which the resin may be spread, and this may cause severe breathing problems.

The following comments apply to poison ivy, poison oak, and sumac.

When does the rash occur?

The allergic skin reaction may start as soon as six hours after exposure but more typically occurs twenty-four to seventy-two hours later. Initially the affected skin is itchy and soon becomes red and raised. Blisters frequently appear later. These often occur in lines or streaks along the course of scratch marks. The rash may continue to erupt for up to two weeks, giving the **mistaken** impression that the rash is being spread by the blister fluid.

Is poison ivy contagious?

Poison ivy dermatitis is **not** contagious and once the initial sap has been washed off **cannot** be spread to other parts of the body or to other people. Not even the blisters are contagious! The delay in the appearance of the later eruptions is probably due to a number of factors including the amount of sap that touches the skin at each location, the varying thickness of the skin, and differences in skin reactivity at various places.

Prevention.

1. Knowing how to identify and then avoiding these plants is the mainstay of prevention of these plant skin rashes.

   Teach your child to recognize these plants.

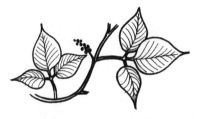

   - **Poison ivy** usually has three leaves that are typically notched ("leaves of three, let them be"). However, there are numerous varieties of poison ivy and some have five leaves! Poison ivy may occur as a vine or shrub. You may not need to go for a walk in the woods to come into contact with poison ivy. You will probably find it in your own backyard!

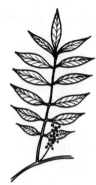

- **Poison sumac** usually has seven to thirteen smooth-edged leaflets. This plant grows in boggy areas in the East and South.

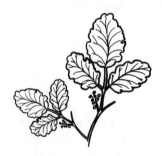

- **Poison oak** occurs in two forms, a low shrub (in the East and South) and a vine (Pacific Coast). The leaves are often notched like those of the oak tree.

  All three plants often have shiny **black spots** on damaged leaves, as the sap of the plant turns black when exposed to the air. The leaves of these plants tend to change color, turning a bright red earlier than most other plants during fall.

2. Your child should wear long-sleeved shirts and long pants when hiking through the woods. This may not be much fun, but the rash of poison ivy is a lot less fun! The poison ivy resin can penetrate clothing and even rubber gloves. When handling poison ivy wear vinyl gloves.

3. You can apply a lotion (for example, *Ivy Block*) to your child's skin before he ventures into poison ivy infested woods. This will help to decrease the severity of the rash but not totally prevent it.

4. Discourage your child from rubbing his eyes after coming into contact with these plants.

5. Take a shower or at least wash all exposed skin after hiking in areas known to contain these plants. Once contact has occurred, the sooner the resin is washed off, the better. It should be washed off with soap and warm water, preferably **within ten minutes.** It is very important to wash under nails, otherwise the resin may spread to other parts of the body by scratching or rubbing. If there has been a long delay, you stand a better chance of removing more resin if the skin is first washed with rubbing alcohol followed by soap and water. Do not use harsh soaps or scrub too vigorously as you are likely to cause even more skin irritation!

6. Change your child's clothes and wash these as well. Handle these clothes with care as you may come into contact with the resin! Boots and boot laces may also become contaminated. It is a good idea to wash the bath towels as well, as they might have become contaminated with the resin.

7. What about desensitization (allergy shots) for poison ivy dermatitis? These have been tried but are **not** very effective.

Treatment of poison ivy rashes.

These comments also apply to the rash of poison oak and sumac.

1. Keep your child as cool as possible. Heat and exercise make any itchy rash worse. Try to stay in a cool environment and wear loose, cool cotton clothes.

2. Cool baths, *Aveeno* compresses and soaks or bland creams or lotions such as *Calamine* lotion will help to decrease the itch.

3. Give your child an oral antihistamine such as diphenhydramine (*Benadryl*). This will help the itch and may even help your child sleep. The newer non-sedating antihistamines will also help to decrease the itch.

4. If your child has an extensive poison ivy reaction and especially if it involves the face or genitalia (not an uncommon location in little boys!), consult your doctor as steroids by mouth may be needed. It is often necessary to continue these oral steroids ten to fourteen days. A common mistake made by many physicians is to prescribe too short a course of steroids. If this is done, the rash will often rebound. Shorter courses of steroids may be effective if started very early in the course of the illness.

5. High-potency topical steroid creams may be effective **if used early** but should **not** be used on the face.

6. Poison ivy is extremely itchy and may be complicated by a **secondary infection** known as impetigo, a skin infection usually due to "staph" or "strep." **Keep your child's nails short** and try to discourage scratching. If the area becomes painful and the area of inflammation continues to spread, your child may need an oral antibiotic or an antibiotic cream. A fever is a definite indication to seek medical care.

WEST NILE FEVER

Refer also to the section on protecting your child against insect and tick bites, page 312.

What is it?

West Nile fever is a **viral** illness that is transmitted by infected mosquitoes. Originally this disease was transmitted by mosquitoes to birds but recently (in the late 1990s), the disease spread to humans and horses.

Where does it occur?

In the United States, West Nile fever was first reported on the East coast but by 2003 had spread as far west as Colorado.

When does it occur?

West Nile fever occurs as an epidemic every **summer and fall.**

What is the incubation period?

Symptoms typically develop three to fourteen days after being bitten by an infected mosquito.

What are the symptoms?

Most people who are bitten by an infected mosquito have **no symptoms** at all! **Some people** have a **mild flu-like**

illness with fever, headache, muscle aches and gastrointestinal symptoms such as nausea and vomiting. Occasionally a rash or enlarged lymph glands may be present.

A very small percentage of people (less than one percent) become **severely ill** with neurological symptoms such as weakness, muscle tremors, and paralysis. Some of these people may die.

What is the risk of catching West Nile Fever?

The risk is extremely **low.** Most mosquitoes do **not** carry the virus. Even if you are bitten by an infected mosquito, your chance of getting the severe form of the disease is less than one percent.

Who gets the severe symptoms?

The severe form of the illness tends to occur in middle-aged or elderly people. It is extremely rare for children to become severely ill from West Nile fever.

How is West Nile fever treated?

There is **no** specific treatment for West Nile fever. Antibiotics are **not** effective against viral infections. The treatment is supportive. Ill patients may require intravenous fluids, help with breathing and specialized medical and nursing care.

How can I prevent West Nile fever?

Even though the risk of acquiring West Nile fever is extremely low, it still makes sense to protect your children and yourself against the disease. This is particularly true for the elderly. You are more likely to get the illness if you spend a lot of time outdoors at the high-risk times.

- During the high risk months, stay indoors at dusk, in the early evening, and dawn. These are the peak times for mosquito bites.

- Wear long-sleeved shirts and long pants when you are outdoors, particularly at peak mosquito biting times.

- Use an effective insect repellent. At the present time this means a repellent containing DEET. (See section on preventing insect and tick bites.) Apply the repellent as often as necessary and wash it off when no longer needed.

- Spray your clothes with permethrin.

- Make sure you have protective screens on windows and doors. Repair defective screens.

- Remove standing water around the house. Empty water from flower pots, buckets, barrels etc. Change the water in bird baths and pet dishes at least once a week. Drill drainage holes in tire swings and keep children's play pools empty when not in use.

342 ◆ PEDIATRIC HEALTH PROBLEMS

LYME DISEASE

Refer also to the section on protecting your child against insects and ticks, page 312.

Lyme disease is caused by a type of bacteria known as a spirochete. This is transmitted to humans when they are bitten by certain types of ticks. In the United States, Lyme disease occurs in three distinct geographic regions:

- The Northeast, extending from southern Maine to Virginia.
- The upper Midwest, especially Wisconsin and Minnesota.
- The West coast, especially northern California.

Lyme disease also occurs in other parts of the world including Canada, Europe, and Asia.

More about the ticks that spread Lyme disease.

In the Northeast, the deer tick is the usual culprit, whereas in the Pacific region, the Western black-legged tick is usually responsible for transmitting the disease. The life cycle of the tick occurs in three stages. These are larva, nymph, and adult. The nymph is usually responsible for transmitting the infection to humans and is very **small**— about the **size of a sesame seed.**

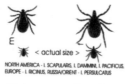

NORTH AMERICA - I. SCAPULARIS, I. DAMMINI, I. PACIFICUS,
EUROPE - I. RICINUS, RUSSIA/ORIENT - I. PERSULCATUS

Male   Female

DEER TICK

The symptoms of Lyme disease.

The symptoms of Lyme disease vary according to the stage of the disease.

- **Early localized disease.** Most people who develop Lyme disease develop a rash which is called **erythema migrans.** This occurs three to thirty-two days (usually seven to fourteen days) after the initial tick bite. It starts as a red spot at the site of the tick bite and enlarges to form a circular lesion, usually with a clear center, often called a "bull's eye." This rash often reaches two to five inches in diameter and may be mistaken for ringworm or eczema. At this time the person will often have flu-like symptoms with fever, chills, headache, and muscle aches.

- **Early disseminated disease.** This occurs some weeks after the initial skin rash and again may include a flu-like illness as well as smaller but similar skin lesions scattered over the body. More significant symptoms include those of meningitis (severe headache and neck stiffness), paralysis of the facial muscles resulting in a facial droop (Bell's palsy), and an irregular or slow heart rate.

- **Late disseminated disease.** This may occur weeks to months after the initial bite. The main manifestation is joint pain (arthritis).

POINTS TO NOTE:

1. Many people do **not** notice the initial tick bite.
2. **Not** all people develop the typical early rash (erythema migrans).
3. **The tick needs to be attached for at least twenty-four hours to transmit the disease.**

How is Lyme disease diagnosed?

The diagnosis of Lyme disease may be very difficult, especially if the typical early rash does not occur and there is no known history of a tick bite. Blood tests are not very helpful in the early stages and may also be confusing and inaccurate later on. The diagnosis is usually based on the typical symptoms occurring in a person who has been in an area where Lyme disease is known to occur.

How is Lyme disease treated?

Lyme disease can be treated very effectively with **antibiotics.** A prolonged course of antibiotics may be needed.

If my child is bitten by a deer tick should he receive a course of antibiotics?

The answer to this question is usually **no.** Even in areas where Lyme disease is common, most ticks are **not** infected. As mentioned above, ticks need to be attached for at least twenty-four hours (and probably as long as forty-eight hours) before they transmit the spirochete that causes Lyme disease. A single dose of *Doxycycline* may be indicated in people over 8 years of age if in a very high risk area and if the tick has been attached for longer than twenty-four hours.

How to prevent Lyme disease.

To prevent Lyme disease you need to prevent tick bites.

- Wear long pants tucked into socks or boots when walking in long grass or the woods. It is easier to see the ticks if you wear light-colored clothing.
- Treat clothes with **permethrin.** (See section on prevention of insect and tick bites.)
- Apply DEET repellent to exposed skin. (See section on prevention of insect and tick bites.)
- After spending time outdoors, do a careful total body inspection for ticks. Look especially carefully in the hair. Remember, the ticks are very small and you will need a good light source to see them.
- If you or your child develops the typical circular rash, seek medical attention.

How to remove an attached tick.

See section on tick bites and tick removal, page 321.

INTO THE WILDERNESS

If you love the outdoors and like to hike, climb, canoe, or camp, you will want to teach your children to enjoy these activities. Start when they are young and you will be able to show them an exciting world that has no television and no computers. Without these distractions, your children will be a captive audience and you will interact on a different level.

Where to go?

- Start close to home when your children are young. We started **very** close to home and after a few nights in a tent in our own backyard, our son was begging to try something more adventurous.
- Choose a location that is familiar to you.
- Be age appropriate. Remember that if you are carrying your child, the distance you travel will depend on your ability and stamina.
- Don't be too ambitious. Consider the skill level of the children.
- Have a backup plan and use it when appropriate.
- Choose a child-friendly destination.

When to go?

- Until your children are experienced, it is better to plan your activities for good weather. Check the forecast before you leave home.

- If you are going to high altitudes, read the chapter on altitude sickness.

Safety.

- Be well prepared.
- Use the best equipment you can afford.
- Take flashlights.
- Give your itinerary to a friend or family member so someone will know where you are.
- A cell phone will be useful if you have a problem and need help.
- Supervise children and set clear guidelines for safe behavior.
- Arrive at campsites in daylight so you can identify potential hazards.
- Teach safe behavior around fires and gas stoves.
- Remember that children are more prone to extremes of temperature.
- Use sunscreen when needed.
- Don't forget insect repellant and mosquito netting.
- Provide each child with a whistle so they can signal for help.
- Bells on the shoes worn by young children will keep parents aware of the children's location.
- Water safety is very important. **Drowning is a common cause of death in childhood.** Wear life jackets when boating. Teach your children how to swim.

Clothing.

- Clothing should be appropriate for the activities and for the weather.
- Layering is a good principle.
- Hats are important. A brim will provide protection from the sun and a warm head covering will prevent heat loss in cold weather.

Shoes.

- Don't try out new shoes on a long hike.
- Take along an extra pair.
- High top shoes will support ankles.
- River shoes protect feet in water.

Food and drink.

- Breast feeding is the most convenient way to feed a baby.
- Powdered formula is convenient if safe water is available.
- Children can carry their own snacks and drinks. Don't wait till they are thirsty or hungry. Encourage them to drink frequently.
- If you will be eating dehydrated food, let your children test these foods at home first.
- S'mores are a treat to enjoy around the camp fire after a day outdoors.

First aid kit.

- Make sure the contents are age appropriate.
- Don't forget sunscreen and insect repellent.

Backpacks and carriers.

- Front carriers are suitable for babies up to twenty pounds.
- Back carriers are suitable for babies seven months and older, when their head and neck are more stable.
- Children can carry a light pack once they are three years of age.
- Children four feet and taller can carry a framed pack. Make sure it is comfortable and fits well.

General points.

- Have fun. Enjoy the journey.
- Be flexible.
- Respect the environment.
- Taking a friend along may ease your child's transition from the electronic world to the wilderness.
- Involve children in planning and preparation.
- Teach children necessary skills and practice them before leaving home. This may include pitching a tent, how to signal when lost, and fire safety.

FOOT CARE

Whether you are hiking in the country, sight-seeing in Europe, or strolling around Disney World, wearing comfortable shoes and having pain-free feet can make or break your trip.

1. Blisters

Blisters are common and frequently occur when hiking or sight-seeing. Pay attention to the following preventative and treatment measures:

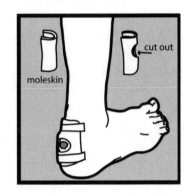

— Before setting out on hiking expeditions or major sight-seeing trips, purchase a blister prevention and repair kit. A well-known brand is *Spenco*. An extra supply of moleskin is also not a bad idea.

— Make sure all footwear is comfortable. Wear shoes or boots that fit properly and have been broken in before your trip or hike starts.

— Wear comfortable socks. When undertaking prolonged hikes, wear two pairs of socks. Ideally, wear a polypropylene sock next to the skin and an outer thicker wool or synthetic sock. Check socks frequently to make sure they are not bunching up. Have spare pairs of clean socks readily available to change into if your socks become wet or damp.

— At rest stops take your socks and shoes off to allow your feet and socks to dry.

— Inspect feet frequently for "hot spots," which are the first sign of blisters. If you see any hot spots, apply some moleskin or *Spenco Second Skin* over the area.

— If a blister develops, do not pop it. Fashion a piece of moleskin or mole foam in a doughnut shape and tape it so that it fits around the inflamed area. This should prevent further friction from occurring.

— If the blister does burst, apply an antibacterial ointment to the area and cover it with a non-adherent dressing. Change this dressing at least every day. If infection does develop (the blister fluid becomes thick and cloudy or the surrounding area becomes very red), start warm soaks when you get back to your base camp or hotel. Continue using the antibacterial ointment. If the surrounding red area increases in size, seek medical care.

For an excellent discussion on the prevention and treatment of blisters, refer to Eric A. Weis' book, *Wilderness and Travel Medicine.*

2. Athletes foot

See section on athlete's foot.

5

Accident Prevention, Injuries, and Emergencies

ACCIDENTS/INJURY PREVENTION

See also: Section on accident prevention while traveling.
Section on fireworks safety.
Section on poisoning.
Section on head injuries
Section on burns

Accidents are the leading cause of death in children one to fifteen years of age! We all worry about our children getting leukemia, brain tumors, Lyme disease, West Nile fever, and other relatively uncommon illnesses. In fact, children are far more likely to die in a motor vehicle accident or from some other preventable accident!

Most accidents are preventable!

Motor vehicle injuries.

Motor vehicle injuries are by far the single greatest cause of death in childhood. You and your child are more likely to survive a motor vehicle accident if you use an appropriate restraint system, whether it is an infant car seat, a booster seat plus seatbelt, or a seatbelt. **You should always set a good example to your child by wearing your seatbelt!**

All infants in the first year of life should be in a rear-facing car seat which is correctly installed. **Eighty percent of child safety seats are installed incorrectly!** Find out how to install your child's car the correct way. You reduce your child's chance of dying or being seriously injured by seventy percent if you use child safety seats correctly. In most communities you should be able to locate an organization that will be able to inspect the installation of your child's car seat to check that you have done this correctly. Often this service is available at your local police station or at a community hospital. Your pediatrician may also be able to advise in this regard.

When your child is one year of age and weighs at least 20 pounds you can switch her to a front-facing car seat. Again, check that it is properly installed! Once she is at least 40 inches tall and weighs about 40 pounds she can progress to a booster seat used together with a seat belt. She should use a booster seat until she fits correctly into the car's combined lap and shoulder belt. The shoulder belt should not cross in front of her face or neck. Parents can find more information about car seat safety by accessing these two websites: http://www.seatcheck.org and http://www.nhtsa.gov. Remember, **the back seat is almost always safer than the front seat!**

Teen drivers and motor vehicle accidents

Teens are even more likely to be injured in car accidents. Driving at night is more dangerous and the greater the number of occupants, the greater the likelihood of an accident. If you add alcohol to the equation you have a recipe for disaster!

Water safety and drowning.

In many parts of the United States drowning is the leading cause of death for children under five years of age. It is also a not uncommon cause of death in teenage males. Here alcohol or swimming in unsafe waters often plays a role. Infants and toddlers may drown in just a few inches of water in a bathtub, bucket, toilet, or outside play pool. **NEVER** leave your young child in the bathtub alone, not even for a few seconds!

Sadly, drowning in swimming pools is also not a rare event. A swimming pool should be surrounded by an appropriate fence on **ALL FOUR SIDES** and have a **gate that locks securely.**

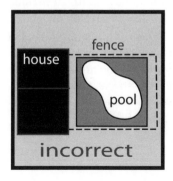
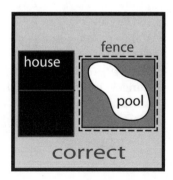

Falls.

Falls often result in significant injury to young children and many visits to the emergency room. These may occur from changing tables, out of cribs, down stairs, or when an inquisitive toddler climbs onto furniture. Do **not** place your child in a mobile baby walker. Accidents related to these have resulted in many deaths!

Burns.

Burns are not only a cause of many childhood deaths but also often result in disfiguring injuries. Tips to avoid burns include:

- Turn down your **hot water settings** to 120° F to 125° F.
- Make sure your home has a number of functioning **smoke alarms.** Replace the batteries every six months, when you turn your clocks forward and back at daylight savings times. Newer **photoelectric smoke detectors** cause fewer false alarms and so are less likely to have their batteries removed!
- Do **not** purchase your own **fireworks.** Rather attend public displays. Fireworks not only can result in serious burns but are also a frequent cause of blindness.
- Keep matches and cigarette lighters in a safe place. Do not leave lighted cigarettes and pipes around. Better still, give up smoking! Not only is secondhand smoke dangerous to your child's health, she is more likely to smoke if you do!

Injury prevention has many other facets to it including:

— **Crib safety.**

— **Firearm safety.** Firearm injuries lead to many tragic deaths in children in the United States. Suicide and homicide due to firearms are significant causes of death in adolescent males!

— **Toy safety.**

— **Playground safety.**

— **Bicycle safety.** Your child is more likely to wear a **bicycle helmet** if you set a good example by wearing yours! Make sure your helmets are fitted correctly.

— **Safety around sports.**

SIDS.

SIDS (sudden infant death syndrome), or crib death, in no way can be classified as an "accident" but there is a preventive aspect to it. SIDS is a significant cause of death in the first year of life.

Ways to avoid SIDS include:

• Place your infant on his back when you put him down to sleep. If he does not like sleeping on his back, sleeping on his side is preferable to sleeping on his tummy. This recommendation applies to healthy infants. Some infants with certain medical conditions may need to be placed on their stomachs to sleep.

• Do not let your infant sleep on soft surfaces.

• Do not put a pillow or blanket in your infants crib.

• Do not smoke when you are pregnant and do not smoke around your baby.

MINOR FALLS AND HEAD INJURIES

Head injuries are extremely common in childhood. Fortunately, most injuries are minor. Infants and toddlers have a relatively large head and limbs that don't always do what they are supposed to do! Toddlers bump their heads frequently as they learn to walk. Usually these bumps are of no consequence and the parent is often more upset by the episode than the child is! Your child will probably cry for a short while after banging his head and may develop a bump (or an "egg"). Most of these bruises will be on the forehead. Over the next day or two, the bruise will darken and a black eye may appear. In fact, the injury often looks more impressive on day two or three than it did in the beginning! Bruises often take up to a week to fade.

The crying will usually cease in ten minutes or less. Many children are a little sleepy after a mild head injury and may even vomit once or twice. This is a common reaction and rarely indicates a more serious problem.

What to do after a minor head injury.

- If your child has broken the skin, clean the abrasion gently with soap and warm water. If your child has a deeper laceration with gaping wound edges, he needs medical attention.

- An older child may be prepared to hold an ice pack against the swelling. Wrap a plastic bag of ice (or a bag of frozen vegetables) in a cloth or towel and apply this to the swelling. It is probably not worth trying to do this if you are dealing with an uncooperative toddler!

- Do **not** give your child ibuprofen (*Advil* or *Motrin*) or aspirin. You may administer a dose of acetaminophen (*Tylenol*) if you feel pain relief is necessary.

- If your child is sleepy, let him sleep. You **don't** have to keep your child awake but you **do** need to keep a close watch on him. If it is nighttime, wake him up when you go to bed and then every four hours or so and check if he is behaving normally. Ask yourself:

  — Does he make good eye contact and appear to be totally "with it?"

  — Can he walk normally?

  — Is he talking normally? You can ask an older child to tell you what his phone number or date of birth is.

  — Are his pupils (the dark spot in the center of the eyes) the same size?

If you are unsure or concerned about any of the answers to the above questions, call your physician. Usually, by the following day your child will have recovered but you will have a few more grey hairs, or perhaps less hair! After a bad fall and especially if brain injury is more likely (see below) it may be necessary to watch your child more closely for another day or night.

WHEN TO CONSULT A
MEDICAL PROFESSIONAL

- If your child **vomits more than two times.**
- If it is **difficult to rouse** your child or he becomes **unconscious.**
- If your child has a **persistent headache** that is becoming **more severe.**
- If an older child is **not behaving, walking, or talking normally.** Confusion, slurred speech, persisting dizziness, clumsiness, or difficulty walking are definitely reasons to seek immediate medical care.
- If your child's **pupils are unequal in size.**
- If your child's **vision** becomes **blurred** or he sees double.
- If your child **remains fussy, irritable, and inconsolable.** These symptoms, as well as changes in eating or nursing, may be the only signs of a problem in a younger child. Most children do not cry for longer than ten minutes after a minor head injury!
- If your child has **blood or watery fluid coming out of one or both ears or his nose.**
- If your child has a **seizure.**
- If, over the following days, your child loses balance easily, seems to regress, loses interest in favorite toys or activities, or his school work deteriorates.

When children are more likely to have brain injuries after a seemingly minor head injury:

— **The younger the child, the more vulnerable the brain.** Children below two years of age and especially those in the first three months of life.

— Falls from **more than three feet in height.**

— **The harder the surface, the more severe the injury.**

— Bumps on the forehead are the least likely to lead to underlying brain injury. Bumps over the temple or the back of the head have a higher chance of being associated with underlying damage.

The above comments on head injury do **NOT** apply to more traumatic injuries such as those involving motor vehicle accidents or falls from great heights or similar severe mechanisms of injury. Nor do they apply to children who have other complicating diseases such as those of the nervous system or bleeding disorders. **Any child under two years of age who has had anything other than a slight bump on the head should be discussed with a physician.**

More severe head injuries.

Your aim should be to **prevent these injuries in the first place:**

Always wear your seat belt. Younger children should be in child safety seats or booster seats.

Never drive under the influence of drugs or alcohol.

Use helmets when appropriate. This includes when riding a bike, a snowmobile, an all-terrain vehicle; when skateboarding, snowboarding, skiing, or riding a horse. Wear a helmet when playing contact sports such as football and ice hockey or when playing baseball and softball. Set a good example for your children by wearing a helmet when you ride a bicycle or partake in activities that may lead to head injuries.

Playground surfaces should be made of shock-absorbing surfaces such as mulch, sand, or rubber.

Keep firearms away from children!

Keep windows and second floor windows of your house fastened. Do not let children play on **balconies.**

NEVER SHAKE YOUR BABY!

SPINE, NECK, AND BACK INJURIES

Spinal injury should be suspected with any severe head injury from trauma such as may occur in a motor vehicle accident, or a fall from a height. Spine and spinal cord injuries are especially common in diving accidents as well as in accidents in sports such as football, biking, horse riding, mountaineering, and skiing.

If the person is conscious and cooperative, tell him not to move until his head, neck, and back have been stabilized. If the victim is unconscious, check that he is breathing adequately. If not, you should check his airway. You may need to gently straighten the head and neck to maintain an open airway.

Whenever a person has sustained an injury that may cause a neck or spinal cord injury, **assume that injury is present and take precautions to prevent damage to the spinal cord.** Do **not** move the victim or elevate the head or neck unless the victim is in life-threatening danger. **Get help.** If you have to move the victim, **roll the person like a log:** roll the body as a single unit, taking care to keep the head, neck, and spine in a straight line. To do this safely in an older child or adult requires the help of at least two other people. To transport the victim, you will need to use a litter or backboard. Place the litter alongside the victim and roll the victim like a log on to the litter. One person will need to cradle the head and neck and give commands to the other people assisting so that all movements are coordinated. It is crucial to support the head during this rolling motion and **keep the head, neck, back, and spine all in a straight line.** Pad and secure the victim with strips of cloth or tape.

Spinal cord injuries are common with head injuries and one should always assume they are present until they have been excluded by x-rays.

POISONING

As children acquire new skills, they expose themselves to new dangers. By six months of age most infants can reach out and grasp objects. These objects go straight to their mouths! By nine months of age, babies have a pincer grip and can pick up small objects between their forefinger and thumb. Around this age they are also becoming more mobile and starting to explore the world. The dangers of accidental poisoning and the risks of choking increase daily and persist throughout the toddler and early childhood years!

Children can ingest a variety of potentially toxic substances. These include both over the counter and prescription medications, household cleaning products, pesticides, plants, gasoline and kerosene, and paints and solvents, to name just a few. Medications that may seem innocuous in small doses, such as acetaminophen (*Tylenol*) and prenatal iron tablets, may be fatal in large doses!

When a parent discovers that her child has ingested a potentially dangerous substance, the parent's natural reaction is to want their child to vomit it out. This may not always be wise! Substances such as strong acids (such as toilet bowl cleaner), or strong alkalis (such as drain cleaner and many detergents) are likely to cause just as much damage coming up as going down! Gasoline and kerosene are more likely to cause a chemical pneumonia if vomiting is induced.

The United States is fortunate in that it has many superb poison centers. These collectively handle over one million accidental ingestions and potential poisonings a year. Fortunately death from poisoning is becoming increasingly rare in the United States. This is due to a combination of factors, the most important being the introduction of child-resistant containers and safer medications as well as increasing public awareness of the dangers of poisoning.

Prevention of poisoning.

Medications

- Keep all medications, including vitamins, out of sight and out of reach. Store them high up and in a locked closet.
- Always secure child-resistant closures in the locked position after use.
- Never transfer a medication from its original container to another.
- Dispose of all unused or no longer needed medicines safely.
- Never refer to medications as candy.

Household products

- Store potentially dangerous products in locked cabinets, preferably high up. Be particularly careful with bleach, drain cleaners, and similar extremely toxic materials.
- Never transfer these substances from their original containers.

In the garage, basement or garden shed

- Store gasoline, kerosene, paint thinners, varnishes in secure containers, locked up and out of reach.
- Never pour these substances into cups, soda bottles or other containers. Even you may forget what that soda bottle contains!
- Store pesticides and fertilizers safely.

Keep the poison center phone number close to the telephone.

The universal number for contacting poison control center in the United States is (800) 222-1222.

Children are often poisoned in someone else's home, so be especially vigilant when visiting relatives and friends. Grandmother's sleeping tablets or blood pressure medicine may look particularly colorful and appealing! People who are not accustomed to having young children around may not be quite as careful about keeping potentially toxic substances in a safe place.

Treatment of poisoning.

- Don't panic!
- Take the substance away from your child. If there is still some poison in your child's mouth, get her to spit it out or remove it with your fingers.
- Look for any obvious, immediate effects such as burns of the lips, redness around the mouth or drooling.
- Contact the poison control center.
- Do **not** induce vomiting until you have discussed this with the poison control center.
- Watch out for side effects such as drooling, drowsiness, retching, stomach cramps, and behavior changes. Call 911 if your child becomes excessively drowsy, unconscious, has breathing difficulties, jerking movements, or seizures. If your child does become unconscious or has a seizure before medical help can be reached, position your child on his side with his head lower than the rest

of his body so that should he vomit, he will not inhale what he threw up. Be alert for breathing difficulties.

• Take the poison, medicine container, or a sample of the ingested material with you to the emergency room. If your child has vomited and you do not know what he ingested, take the vomited material with you to the hospital.

The use of ipecac in the treatment of poisoning

Ipecac syrup is a liquid that induces vomiting. Your pediatrician or family practitioner may have recommended that you purchase ipecac syrup and keep it in the home so that you can administer it to your child in the event that she ingests a poisonous substance or a potentially dangerous medication. In 2003, the American Academy of Pediatrics changed its recommendation that you keep ipecac in the home and use it routinely as a poison treatment intervention. This was done for a number of reasons which included the fact that ipecac is not always very effective, it is sometimes inappropriate to administer it and inducing vomiting is frequently not necessary.

There may be circumstances where it is advisable to have ipecac available for the treatment of poisoning. Such a circumstance would be the traveling family that does not have easy access to a poison control center. Families traveling to malarial areas may be carrying chloroquine with them to prevent malaria. If an inappropriately large amount of chloroquine is ingested by a young child the consequences may be fatal! Prompt administration of ipecac may be life-saving.

There may be other occasions when you do not have access to a poison center or medical care. In this case check the container that contained the substance. There may be instructions to guide you on how to take care of the ingestion. Remember, sometimes these guidelines are out of date so it is always better to contact a poison center if possible. If you have ipecac with you, you may decide to use it. Give 3 tsp or 1 tbsp (15ml) followed by a glass of juice or water.

NEVER ADMINISTER IPECAC IF . . .

— The ingested substance is a strong acid or a strong alkali.
— The ingested substance is gasoline, kerosene, or a similar volatile material.
— The victim is very drowsy or unconscious.

Remember, no matter where you are it is always better to prevent these sorts of accidents!

> **Keep medicines and toxic substances in a SAFE PLACE IN A SECURE CONTAINER!**

WOUND CARE—MINOR CUTS, SCRAPES (ABRASIONS), BRUISES, AND BLEEDING

All children have falls and minor accidents from time to time. Many of these injuries can be handled at home and do not require professional medical attention.

Guidelines.

1. **Remain calm.** Your child will pick up cues from your behavior. The more upset you act, the more frightened he will become. Often, the louder your child cries, the less severe the injury! The wound often looks worse than it is, especially if there is brisk bleeding. Sometimes, relatively minor injuries are associated with a lot of bleeding. This is likely to happen if the injury is on the scalp, where there is a large supply of blood vessels close to the surface. Abrasions or superficial (first degree) burns are very painful but not very serious.

2. **Clean the wound properly.** If possible, hold the affected area under running water and clean the wound thoroughly. If this is not possible, clean the area with soap and water. In the case of animal or human bites, hold the affected area under running water for at least five to ten minutes. A small amount of bleeding will do no harm and may actually help remove bacteria and debris.

3. When the wound is thoroughly cleaned, apply an antiseptic or antibacterial ointment and cover it with clean gauze and fasten it with tape. At times, all that is needed is a band aid.

4. If the wound is still bleeding after you have cleaned it, place clean gauze directly over the area and apply firm pressure. If you do not have clean gauze, use a clean handkerchief or clean cloth. Elevating the affected part, for example, the foot or the hand, will also help to control the bleeding. If the bleeding continues, medical care should be sought.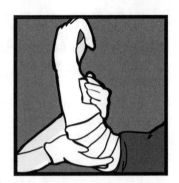

5. If the wound is deep and gaping, your child will probably need stitches— seek medical attention. If you are traveling and away from home and medical help is not easily accessible, you can try to pull the edges of the wound together using a *Steri-strip* or a butterfly band aid. You can make your own butterfly band aid from adhesive tape.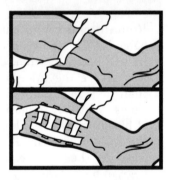

6. Your child may need a **tetanus shot,** especially if he is not fully immunized or the wound is contaminated with debris. Most children get tetanus immunizations as part of their routine childhood immunizations.

7. In the case of an animal bite, your child might need protection against **rabies.** Contact your physician for guidance. In certain parts of the world, especially Asia, animal bites have a much higher risk of rabies. (See section on rabies, page 382.)

8. It is important to **keep the wound clean and dry as it heals.** Many wounds will become infected if a band aid or other dressing is left on for too long. **Replace the band aid or dressing on a daily basis.** Clean the wound every day and allow it to air dry.

9. Watch out for **signs of infection** which include redness and swelling that spreads outward from the wound, red streaks spreading up the limb from the wound site, worsening pain, or a fever. Wounds of the hands and feet may be deeper than they appear and infection can spread rapidly in these sites. Most puncture wounds are often deeper than they appear and are likely to become infected. Puncture wounds of the hands or feet should be assessed by a medical professional.

BURNS

Each year, more than two million people in the United States suffer from burn injuries. Children, especially boys, make up the majority of these burn victims. The most common burn encountered is a **scald** due to hot liquids or steam. This usually happens **in the kitchen or bathroom.** Burns may also be caused by flames, chemicals, electricity, or radiation. **Sunburn** is the most frequent cause of a radiation burn. If sunburn is the problem, refer to the section on sunburn.

> The skin is the largest organ in the body and its thickness varies greatly according to the location. The skin of the palms and soles may be up to ten times thicker than that of the eyelids. The thinner the skin, the greater the sensitivity to heat. Burns may also be associated with other injuries including smoke **inhalation** damage to the lungs.

If your child has suffered a severe burn injury, seek medical care immediately!

Burns are classified according to:

- **Size.** The larger the burned area the more severe the consequences. The palm of the victim's hand is equal to about one percent of the entire skin surface area. Even a superficial (first degree) burn of ten percent can have serious consequences in a child!

- **Depth.** Heat burns can be classified into three degrees. This classification is not always easy to do and often has to be revised a day or two after the burn has taken place.

  — **First degree.** This is fortunately the most common and is characterized by superficial redness and pain. The skin will turn white when you press on it. The skin often peels within the next two to three days and is totally healed by one week. Sunburn is usually a first degree burn.

— **Second degree or partial thickness burns.** Characterized by deeper redness, more severe pain, swelling, and **blistering.** Depending on their depth, these burns may take up to four weeks to heal. If these burns become infected, they may convert into a third degree or full thickness burn. Most less-severe scalds are second degree burns and usually take seven to fourteen days to heal.

— **Third degree.** Here the burned area is leathery and either white or charred. The burned skin itself is not painful but the surrounding area may be. These burns will require skin grafting.

NOTE: Second and third degree burns readily become infected by bacteria.

• **Location.** Burns of the **face, hands, feet,** and **genital area** have complications out of proportion to their size and should **always be assessed by a medical professional.**

What to do if your child gets a burn.

• Remove your child from the heat source.
• Remain calm.
• Immerse the burned area in cold water, or if this is not possible, cover the area with a cloth soaked in cold water. This will not only limit the burn size but also provide some pain relief.
• Do **not** apply butter, oil, or sprays to the burn. Benzocaine and other local anesthetic sprays may lead to sensitization.

- Give your child an analgesic such as ibuprofen (*Advil* or *Motrin*) or acetaminophen (*Tylenol*). In the case of burns, ibuprofen is superior to acetaminophen and if administered within 4 hours of a burn may limit extension of the burn.

- After the initial cool water soak, for first degree burns apply a skin care product such as aloe vera. For second degree burns apply either aloe vera or an antibiotic ointment and cover the burn with a non-stick dressing such as *Telfa* if you have this available. Keep it in place with gauze and tape. An ideal cream for deeper second degree burns is *Silvadene,* which is available only by prescription.

- Do **not** pop the blisters.

WHEN TO SEEK MEDICAL CARE

— If the burn covers an area larger than the palm of your child's hand.

— With any burn of the face, hands, feet, or genital area.

— If the burn is anything other than a first degree burn. The degree of the burn may be difficult to assess. If you are unsure, seek medical care.

— If the burn becomes infected. Signs of infection may include:
  - Wound discharge that is green or yellow.
  - Increasing pain at the burn site after a day or two.
  - Increased swelling or redness of the skin surrounding the burn.
  - A fever.

— If your child gets an electrical burn.

— If your child has a second or third degree burn he may require a **tetanus shot.**

Follow-up care.

- Burns other than first degree burns will require dressing changes once a day. Soak the burned area in cool water for fifteen minutes, allow to air dry, and then apply an antibiotic ointment. Cover with a non-stick dressing such as *Telfa,* and keep it in place with gauze and tape. It is a good idea to give your child a suitable analgesic such as acetaminophen or ibuprofen one hour **before** you change the dressing.

- Be on the lookout for secondary infection (described above).

- Once the burn has healed, soften the area by rubbing in vitamin E cream.

- Be extra careful to avoid sunburn to the area for at least one year.

Electrical burns.

1. Do not touch the victim until the current has been turned off or the source of the current has been removed with an implement such as a wooden broomstick, which does not conduct electricity.

2. If the victim is unconscious, call 911 and begin CPR if necessary.

3. If the victim is otherwise OK, treat the burn like other heat burns by immersing the burned part in cold water if possible.

4. Use pain medicine as necessary.

5. Seek medical care.

NOTE:
Electrical burns may appear to be very minor on the sur-
face, but **serious deep tissue injury** may have occurred.
Internal injuries may also be present.

PREVENTION OF BURNS

Most burns can be prevented!

— Prevent sunburn by taking appropriate precautions.
  (See section on sunburn.)

— Use smoke alarms in your home. Do not disconnect
  these alarms! Replace the batteries twice a year.

— Do not leave lighted cigarettes, matches, or cigarette
  lighters around. Better still, give up smoking!

— Be careful in the kitchen. Turn pot handles to the
  side or back of the stove. Preferably use the back
  burners of the stove.

— Do **not** hold your child on your lap when drinking
  hot beverages.

— Keep your hot water temperature between 120 to
  125 degrees Fahrenheit. Check the water temperature before putting your child in the bath.

— **Be especially careful when using curling irons.**
  These are extremely hot and cause deep burns very
  quickly.

— **Don't leave a hot iron on the ironing board.** They
  are too unstable!

— Don't leave burning candles within your toddler's
  reach!

— Keep caustic chemicals (strong alkalis and acids) in a safe place and in secure containers.

— Put covers on electrical outlets.

— If your car has been standing in the sun, check the temperature of your child's car seat before putting her in it. Hot buckles can burn an infant's or toddler's sensitive skin.

FOREIGN BODY IN THE NOSE

It is not unusual for children to put things other than their fingers up their noses! Objects that commonly find their way into the nose are popcorn kernels, buttons, beads, eraser tips, and candy. More potentially dangerous objects that are put in the nose are small batteries such as camera or watch batteries. These can cause erosions of the nasal septum (the part of the nose that separates the two nostrils).

If your child confesses that he has put something up his nose it is wise to seek medical help immediately. Your doctor may be able to remove it fairly easily but occasionally this may have to be done by an ENT (ear, nose, and throat) surgeon under anesthesia.

You may be able to see the object in the nose and if it is protruding you may be able to remove it yourself. However, do **not** try to get it out yourself if you cannot easily get a hold of it as you may push it in deeper. Do **not** try to push it in deeper hoping it will land up in the victim's throat and be coughed out or spat out! If you do this it may be aspirated into the windpipe or lungs. Rarely, a cooperative older child may be able to force it out of his nose by blowing his nose or by sneezing.

Sometimes a child does not tell the parent what he has done and the parent gradually becomes aware over time that the child has bad breath and a nasty discharge out of **one** nostril!

Rarely, a child who has put an object up his nose will swallow it, in which case there is usually nothing to be concerned about unless it is a battery or a sharp object. The major concern with a foreign body up the nose is that it will be aspirated into the airway or lungs. If your child has a choking episode, medical care should be sought immediately! If your child is in severe distress, you may have to perform the Heimlich maneuver or some similar age-appropriate maneuver. (See section on choking, page 414.)

REASONS TO SEEK MEDICAL CARE

- A foreign body in the nose which cannot be easily and immediately removed.
- A persistent foul-smelling discharge from one nostril.
- A choking episode or breathing difficulty in a child who was known to be playing with small objects.
- If you suspect your child may have swallowed a potentially dangerous object such as a camera battery, watch battery, or a sharp object

---

EYE INJURIES AND FOREIGN BODIES IN THE EYE

See section on eye problems, page 245.

KNOCKED OUT TOOTH

Dental injuries are common in childhood, one of the more common being a knocked out tooth.

- If a young child knocks out a **"baby" or milk tooth,** do not attempt to replace it.

- If your child knocks out a **permanent (adult) tooth** this should be replaced as soon as possible. Do **not** touch the root end. Rinse the tooth *gently* under running water and replace it. Do **NOT** scrub or attempt to clean the tooth too vigorously. If you are unable to replace the tooth put it in a glass of water or milk and seek dental attention right away. The sooner the tooth is replaced in the gum socket the more likely it is to take hold and survive. Even if you have successfully replaced the tooth, consult your dentist as the tooth may need to be splinted. Your child may also need an antibiotic.

- If the tooth is only partially dislodged and is just sticking out of its socket farther than normal, push it back in until it is in its normal position and seek medical or dental attention.

- After dental trauma, your child should be on a liquid or soft diet until the tooth has healed.

- If the tooth cannot be found, your child may need to be checked because the tooth may have been inhaled. If this is the case your child will probably be coughing or be in respiratory distress. A chest x-ray may be needed to make sure this did not happen. If the tooth has been swallowed, apart from the fact that your child has lost a tooth, there is no need to be concerned.

- To control bleeding from the gum apply pressure with clean gauze or a clean cloth. Bleeding will usually stop if pressure is applied for long enough. As with bleeding in other locations, you may need to apply constant pressure for five to ten minutes.

BITES

Bites not only cause immediate tissue damage but also carry the risk of infection and rabies. Human bites are the bites most likely to become infected, followed by cat bites and then dog bites. Cat bites may look very minor but infected material is often injected deeply into the tissues.

The most important treatment of any bite is vigorous cleaning of the wound as soon as possible. This is best done by holding the affected area under running water for at least five to ten minutes. Contact your doctor for further treatment—such as tetanus shots, rabies prevention, antibiotics, and/or suturing if needed. This will depend on the bite size, location, and likelihood of infection. For crush injuries, splinting and elevation of the affected extremity may be indicated. **It is especially important to seek medical care for bites involving the face and puncture wounds of the hands and feet.**

If your child has been bitten by a wild animal or a domestic animal that you don't know, rabies prophylaxis may be needed. (See section on rabies, page 382.)

RABIES

Rabies and rabies prevention are still significant public health issues in the United States. Rabies in humans is fortunately rare because of prophylactic measures after animal bites and because of control of rabies in domestic animals. It is also a major medical issue in developing countries, with up to 100,000 human deaths worldwide annually!

The culprits.

In the United States, the animals that usually spread rabies are raccoons, skunks, foxes and bats. Raccoons are the number one cause. In developing countries, the most frequent cause of rabies is dog bites.

Prevention.

1. Immunize your pets against rabies.
2. Use caution around animals you do not know, even domestic ones.
3. Avoid physical contact with strays and wild animals, whether dead or alive.
4. Do not attempt to domesticate wild animals, especially raccoons.
5. Tightly secure garbage can lids and make them less accessible to prowling dogs, raccoons, and skunks.

Remember, in developing countries, dogs are the number one cause of rabies. Caution your children about petting dogs in third world countries, especially in Asia.

Domestic pets such as white rats, hamsters, and mice do **not** carry rabies. Squirrel bites would be very unlikely to lead to rabies. If there is any doubt, contact your doctor or local public health authorities. Be especially wary of **bats:** your child does **not** have to be bitten by a bat to get rabies. Rabies may be transmitted via bat urine or other bat secretions which enter through a child's mucous membranes such as the eye or mouth. If there is any doubt about your child's exposure to a bat while sleeping, contact your doctor or local health authorities.

Treatment.

Initial treatment of any animal bite includes **extensive cleansing,** as mentioned in the section under animal bites, followed by further wound care as necessary. Your child may need tetanus prevention as well as antibiotics. Your doctor will then determine whether a course of rabies shots is necessary.

NOTE:
If you intend to visit and stay in an area where there is a high incidence of rabies, consider immunizing your children against rabies before you depart. This may be important if you are planning a **long stay** in a lesser-developed country where rabies is common. Discuss this with your doctor prior to your travels.

HEAT-RELATED ILLNESS— HEAT SYNCOPE, HEAT CRAMPS, HEAT EXHAUSTION, AND HEAT STROKE

There are other causes for elevated temperatures besides the fever that occurs with infections. Heat-related illnesses include heat syncope, heat cramps, heat exhaustion, and heat stroke. Unlike the fever that occurs with infection (which is the body's normal way of fighting infection), heat related illnesses are abnormal and may be very serious. Each year, heat stroke is responsible for more than 400 deaths in the United States!

- **Heat syncope.** It is not unusual for a person who has been standing for a long time in a hot environment to feel lightheaded and faint.

- **Heat cramps** usually follow strenuous exercise such as cycling on a hot day when the body has been depleted of salts and water. The muscles most commonly involved are the calves, the thighs, and the abdominal muscles. People with heat cramps are generally **alert,** have a normal temperature, and complain of muscle cramps. Treatment is to rehydrate with salt-containing fluids such as sports drinks or electrolyte solutions. Muscle cramps may also occur in tandem with heat exhaustion and heat stroke, in which case more aggressive treatment will be needed.

- **Heat exhaustion.** A child with heat exhaustion will be very fatigued and complain of headache, dizziness, or nausea. He may be mildly confused and vomit. He will sweat excessively. The skin is often cool and clammy. Usually the temperature is elevated but it may be normal. If he remains in the hot environment and without fluids, he may progress to the next stage of heat illness known as heat stroke.

• **Heat stroke** is the final and most severe stage of heat illness. People with heat stroke are usually **very confused** and the body temperature is usually markedly elevated, often to 105 degrees Fahrenheit or higher. The skin is often dry. As heat stroke worsens, the level of consciousness deteriorates; the person may have a seizure or lapse into a coma. Shock frequently develops. **Heat stroke is extremely dangerous and is a medical emergency.**

People of all ages may get heat-related injuries but certain groups are particularly prone to develop these problems:

➤ Infants and young children.

Infants and young children do not sweat as readily as adults and have greater fluid requirements relative to their size. They are more prone to dehydration and heat-related illness. They also tend to be more active and are often "too busy" to stop to drink! Infants have an immature temperature regulation system, which contributes to the problem. Infants may suffer from heat exhaustion or heat stroke when they are over bundled or over swaddled, especially if they have mild infections associated with a fever. A very serious and preventable cause of heat-related illness in infants and young children is being left in a closed car. Temperatures in the car on hot days may exceed 150 degrees Fahrenheit. Even a few minutes at these temperatures may be fatal!

➢ Older children.

Older children are prone to heat illness when they exercise on very hot days, especially if it is humid and they have not yet acclimatized to the heat. Young athletes are especially likely to develop heat stroke if they do not drink sufficient fluid or if they are overweight. This type of heat illness may occur even in very fit adults who are dehydrated and exercising on hot days.

➢ The elderly.

The elderly may develop heat exhaustion or heat stroke without exercising if exposed to high environmental temperatures for several days, as occurs during heat waves.

Treatment of heat-related illness.

The treatment of the **less severe forms of heat-related illness** includes moving to a cooler environment (such as the shade), removing excess clothing, and taking in plenty of fluids. Wetting the victim with cool water or fanning is very beneficial. If a person has heat cramps, give salt-containing fluids such as *Pedialyte* or sports drinks. If these are not available, drinking water to which a small amount of salt has been added (¼ tsp of salt to 1 quart of water) is a good alternative. Do **NOT** give the victim salt tablets. If the person is confused or vomiting, then **immediate medical care** should be sought. Do **not** administer aspirin, ibuprofen, or acetaminophen as they do **not** help this condition and may be harmful.

As mentioned above, **heat stroke** is a medical emergency and may be fatal. Activate emergency medical services (call 911). While waiting for medical help to arrive you should do the following:

— Move the victim to a cooler area.

— Remove all the clothing down to the underwear. Young children and infants should have all their clothing removed.

— Sprinkle or spray the victim with cool water or repeatedly apply wet towels or cloths.

— Fan the victim.

— Place ice packs, cold compresses, or chemical ice packs around the neck, the armpits, the groin, and the scalp.

— Do **not** force the victim to drink if he is confused or comatose.

— Do **not** give the patient aspirin, ibuprofen, or acetaminophen.

Prevention of heat-related illness

• **Infants and young children should not be overdressed, particularly if they have a fever or infection.** The fever associated with an infection does not cause brain damage and is seldom cause for worry. However, if an infant who is ill and has a fever is overdressed or is in a warm environment, his temperature may reach dangerous levels. This may lead to severe medical problems, including brain damage.

• Never leave children in hot cars, even for short periods.

Prevention of exercise-related heat injury.

- **Gradual acclimatization** to hot weather is important. Expose your child to hotter temperatures for a few minutes longer each day. Increase activity intensity and duration a little each day. Do not let your child exercise vigorously in hot and humid weather until this acclimatization has taken place.

- Do not let your child exercise at the hottest times of the day. At the beginning of the season, plan activities for the early morning or evening when temperatures are cooler. As your child becomes acclimatized to the warmer weather and is fitter, then activities can take place in hotter and more humid weather and exercise periods can last longer.

- Dress children in **lightweight and light-colored clothing,** which allows their skin to breathe and allows them to sweat adequately.

- Drink **extra fluids** before beginning exercise. Children should stop frequently (every twenty minutes) for drinks of water or sports drinks. **Children should <u>not</u> wait until they are thirsty to drink.** If your child waits until he is thirsty to drink he is far more likely to become dehydrated and develop heat-related illness. Adolescents at football practice may want to appear "macho" and say they do not need to drink. **Everyone** at the practice **must** drink! Avoid caffeine-containing drinks, as these increase urine output.

- Children also need to have **frequent breaks in the shade** to cool off. This is especially important for overweight children. Any child who appears to be very fatigued, flushed, dizzy or who seems less alert than usual, should be called off the field immediately, be taken to a cooler location, and given fluids. Such a child should be closely watched.

- All children should try to get fit **before** the sports season starts. This is even more important for overweight children as they are particularly prone to heat exhaustion and heat stroke.

- **Vacationing and heat illness.**
  Vacationers are particularly prone to heat illness. It is not unusual to be at sub-zero temperatures in the Northeast on one day and be in a hot and humid climate the next! These measures may help you avoid heat-related illness and ruining your vacation.

  — Schedule activities for early and late in the day when it is cooler.

  — Increase your sun exposure gradually.

  — Wear a hat and apply sunscreen if out in the sun.

  — Wear loose-fitting, cool, cotton clothes.

  — Drink plenty of fluids.

  — Limit your caffeine and alcohol intake.

COLD RELATED INJURY— FROST NIP, FROST BITE, AND HYPOTHERMIA

Just as children are more prone to heat injury than adults, so are they more likely to suffer from cold injury. The younger and smaller the child, the greater the risk. Children have a large surface area relative to their body weight, as well as a relatively large head from which they lose heat. They also have thinner skin which loses heat more easily, less subcutaneous fat, and fewer energy reserves. All this is compounded by immaturity and poor judgment. The elderly are also prone to the development of hypothermia.

If the body temperature drops to 95° Fahrenheit or lower, this is known as **hypothermia.** If just part of the body freezes, this is known as **frostbite.** Hypothermia and frostbite often occur together.

Hypothermia.

This occurs when the body temperature drops. It is classified as mild, moderate, or severe (deep) hypothermia. The more severe forms are extremely serious and may be fatal! The signs of mild hypothermia may be very subtle and it frequently "sneaks up" gradually and insidiously.

Signs of *mild* hypothermia include:

- Shivering.
- Cold, blue, and mottled extremities.
- Numb hands and feet; stiff muscles which lead to clumsy and uncoordinated movements and stumbling.

- Lethargy, apathy, weakness, confusion, and poor judgment.
- Slurred speech.

As the hypothermia becomes more severe, the person will become more and more confused and irrational. With severe hypothermia, shivering ceases, the heart rate slows, and the person will lapse into unconsciousness. This is a medical emergency.

Frostnip and frostbite.

The areas most likely to be affected by both frostnip and frostbite are the fingers, toes, cheeks, and the tips of the ears and nose. **All but the most minor degree of cold injury requires medical attention.**

Frostnip is the mildest form of cold injury and only involves the superficial layers of the skin. The affected area is cold and white. Initially it may be painful, but later it becomes slightly numb but still has some sensation. As the area is warmed, it turns red and the person may feel a tingling sensation ("pins and needles"). Frostnip is totally reversible and is cured by warming. There is **no** permanent damage, but if not treated early and adequately it will progress to the more severe frostbite.

Frostbite is more severe than frostnip, as ice crystals actually form in the tissues and cause damage.

Frostbite is classified, according to the depth of the freezing injury, into superficial and deep frostbite. Early on it may be extremely difficult to differentiate between different degrees of frostbite.

— *Superficial frostbite* affects the skin and the tissues immediately below the skin. The affected area usually has a pale and waxy appearance but there may be surrounding redness. The area will feel doughy and thickened. It will be numb. With thawing, blisters that contain a clear fluid may form. If the injury is slightly deeper the fluid may be milky.

— *Deep frostbite* is an extremely serious injury extending into the underlying tissues and may involve tendons, muscles, and sometimes bone. The entire area will have a woody feel with no sensation. If blisters form they are filled with a purple fluid.

As frostbite is warmed and thawed, the affected area often becomes red, blotchy, and very swollen. **Thawing is often accompanied by extreme pain.** The deeper degrees of frostbite may lead to death of the tissues and amputation may be necessary.

Prevention of cold injury.

Most cold injuries are preventable. Remember, hypothermia can occur in all seasons and **not** only in the winter months.

When planning outdoor activities where cold injury is possible, consider the following.

A) Clothing

• Dress your child in **layers.** Air gets trapped between layers and provides extra insulation. Layering also allows one to remove clothing as one gets warmer and add a layer as one gets colder. Ideally, the layer closest to the skin should be made of a synthetic fiber such as polypropylene or polyester which wicks perspiration away from the skin. The *middle layer* provides insulation and some protection from the outside and may be made of wool, fleece, or cotton. This layer also absorbs some of the moisture from the inner layer. The *outer layer* should provide insulation as well as be wind- and water-resistant. This layer should also allow some ventilation so that sweat may evaporate.

- Children should wear **hats.** The younger the child, the greater the heat loss from the head. A person may lose up to eighty percent of her body heat from the head and neck. A warm hat, a warm scarf, and ear muffs are essential!

- **Gloves or mittens.** Mittens provide greater protection from the cold but with loss of dexterity. On very cold days it is a good idea to use silk or polypropylene **glove linings.**

- **Foot protection and boots.** Boots should fit well so as not to restrict the circulation. Just as having two layers on the hands is a good idea, wearing two pairs of socks will help keep the toes and feet warm. Always have spare dry pairs of socks available. Change socks frequently so that the feet remain dry. Cold feet lead to frostbite, clumsiness, and misery!

- **Remove** underlying layers of clothes as your child heats up with activity. Being too warm leads to sweating. Clothing gets damp and this leads to chilling as one cools down. **Add** these layers back on as your child cools down again.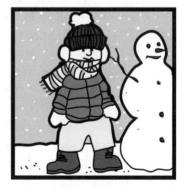

B) Fluids and nutrition

- **Fluids.** One is more susceptible to cold injury if one is dehydrated. Encourage your child to drink even if he is not thirsty. Avoid caffeine-containing drinks. Adults **MUST** avoid alcohol! Urine color, usually a good indication of the state of hydration, should be a **light** yellow.

- **Calories** are also needed to help ward off the cold. Frequent high-carbohydrate snacks provide instant energy. If camping outdoors at night, eat foods that contain fat and protein to provide your body with energy all night.

C) Environmental conditions

Use common sense.

- Do not allow your child to go outside on extremely cold days. Make sure your child is adequately and appropriately dressed even on days that are not that cold but where wind chill is possible.

- Remember, **wind** and **wetness** make cold injury much more likely! Your child should not be outside if the **wind chill index** is below 10 degrees Fahrenheit.

- Limit time spent outdoors on cold days. Do **not** wait until your child is chilled before getting him indoors!

- Suspect hypothermia if a child who has been playing outside in the cold is irritable or lethargic or behaving strangely.

Hiking, climbing and camping trips.

- Plan trips carefully, paying due attention to the weather conditions and location.

- Plan ahead. Anticipate changes in the weather and temperature and even on sunny days include a water- and wind-resistant shell, a warm hat, mittens, extra pairs of socks, food, and **adequate fluids.** A space blanket is lightweight and packs easily.

- Hunger, exhaustion, and demoralization all make hypothermia more likely. Plan excursions carefully and sensibly. Don't try to do too much. **Activities should be set at the level of the weakest and slowest participant.** Eat snacks regularly.

- Keep an eye on your companions.

  — Use the "buddy" system to check each others' faces (the nose, ears, and cheeks) for telltale signs of frostbite (redness or white or yellow plaques).

  — Repeatedly assess your companions: Are they drinking enough? Are they becoming irritable, lethargic, irrational, or confused? Do they just want to be left alone? Are they becoming less coordinated?

These signs may all indicate hypothermia. Take action!

Driving in the winter.

- Put blankets, gloves, extra clothes, and some food and water in the car when setting out on winter travel. A cell phone, a flashlight, flares, and a shovel may also turn out to be very useful!

- If you become stranded:

  — Stay inside your car for shelter if it is cold outside.

  — Make sure the snow does not block your car's exhaust pipe.

  — Turn off the engine and anything that consumes energy (lighter, heater, and radio).

— Run the engine and heater for ten minutes every hour.

— Open the window a little now and then. Snuggle together but stretch regularly to keep awake and keep warm.

— If snow starts to bury your car, it is a good idea to make an air hole with an umbrella, a ski, or similar object.

— **Do not drink alcohol!**

Treatment of cold injuries.

The treatment will depend not only on the type or severity of the injury but also on where you are and your proximity to medical help. If you are at home and your child is getting cold, get him to COME INSIDE!

Although hypothermia and frostbite often coexist, **treat the hypothermia first** as this is more likely to be fatal.

Hypothermia

Severe hypothermia is a medical emergency! Although the principles of treatment apply to all degrees of hypothermia, the treatment of the more severe degrees of hypothermia are beyond the scope of this book. If you are in a situation where you can call 911, do this immediately. Prevent further heat loss by *gently* removing wet clothing and covering with layers of dry clothing, blankets, and/or sleeping bags. **Handle the victim very gently!**

For the *milder degrees of hypothermia,* do the following:

• Get the victim out of the cold and wind if possible.

• Remove all wet clothing. Put on dry clothing in layers.

- Cover the victim with warm, dry blankets or put the victim into a sleeping bag. Two sleeping bags are better than one.
- Offer the victim a warm, sweet drink.

Once the victim is out of the cold and you have followed the above directions, shivering will generate heat and raise the body temperature. **If at all possible, do NOT leave a hypothermic person alone!**

Frostbite

- Get out of the cold.
- **Always try to detect and treat frostnip and frostbite early**—as soon as the body part turns numb and white. Older children and adults should try "windmilling" (swinging arms and hands vigorously in a rotary fashion) when their fingers and hands first start getting numb.
- For *mild* frostbite, remove wet clothing (gloves, mittens, boots, and socks) and warm by skin to skin contact. Place hands in the armpits and place cold feet under clothing on somebody else's belly or in an armpit.
- Remove rings, watches, and tight or constrictive clothing that may compromise the circulation as swelling occurs.
- Put on dry gloves or mittens, dry socks, dry boots, and warm clothing.

More severe frostbite will require more intensive treatment. Get medical help if possible! The ideal treatment is rapid thawing accomplished by soaking the affected part in warm water (100 to 108 degrees Fahrenheit). This is not always possible and one often has to allow slow and spontaneous warming if a great distance from warmth and shelter. Once thawing has occurred, **it is essential to prevent refreezing of the affected area.** If this occurs, more damage will result. If one cannot prevent refreezing, it is better not to allow thawing in the first place.

If you are out on the trail or in the mountains and a member of your party gets frostbite of the feet it is OK to let that person walk out with frozen feet. Thawing is likely to take place spontaneously. Again, prevent refreezing. If boots are taken off out on the trail, you stand the risk of not being able to put them back on again!

Remember, frostbite is often associated with hypothermia. Treat hypothermia first!

IMPORTANT DON'TS

- Don't rub frost-bitten tissues. This may lead to further damage! Especially do not rub with snow.
- **Don't allow to refreeze!**
- Don't heat the frost-bitten area in front of the fire or heater. Don't try to warm the frozen area with a blow dryer! You may complicate the injury with a burn!
- Don't break blisters.
- Don't touch cold metal with bare hands!
- Don't handle fuel and super-cooled liquids with bare hands.

SOME INTERESTING FACTS ABOUT COLD INJURIES.

1. **Dehydration** predisposes to hypothermia and frostbite. Keep well hydrated!
2. **Wetness often leads to hypothermia!**
   - This wetness may come from the **outside**—rain, snow or water.

- Wetness may come from the **inside**—sweating leads to damp clothes, leading to conduction of heat away from the body, and finally chilling.
- **Heat is lost twenty-five times faster in water!** If you are out boating and your boat capsizes, you are more likely to survive by clinging on to the overturned hull than by trying to swim to a distant shore through cold waters. This applies even if your clothes are soaked and you are exposed to the rain and wind!

3. **Hypothermia can occur in all seasons, not only in winter!** A person may get dangerous hypothermia even when outside temperatures are 50–60 degrees Fahrenheit if there is wind chill or clothing is damp or inadequate! **The person who sets off on a hike on a sunny day in shorts and a t-shirt and gets caught in the rain is more likely to get hypothermia than the well-prepared skier in the middle of winter.**

For those undertaking more adventurous activities, it is strongly recommended that you read more to learn about cold- and heat-related injuries, first aid in the wilderness, and similar topics. *Wilderness and Travel Medicine* by Eric Weiss or *Wilderness First Aid,* a collaboration between the National Safety Council and the Wilderness Medical Society and published by Jones and Bartlett publishers, are excellent sources for further information. The truly adventurous are advised to go on one of the survival courses offered by the Wilderness Medical Society.

FIREWORK SAFETY AND INJURIES

Every year, particularly around the 4th of July, children are injured by fireworks. Almost 10,000 people visit the emergency room each year with injuries caused by fireworks. Over 1,000 of these injuries involve the eyes. In fact, **fireworks are a significant cause of blindness!**

- Burns are the most common injury due to fireworks.

- Bottle rockets cause the greatest number of eye injuries.

- Sparklers frequently cause eye injuries. They can reach temperatures of 1,800 degrees Fahrenheit, hot enough to melt gold!

- Bystanders are more often injured than those who operate the fireworks!

Prevention of fireworks injuries.

Leave it to the professionals. Do not set off fireworks yourself. Don't be around amateurs setting off fireworks. That is all you need to know!

First aid management of fireworks injuries.

- For burns, see section on burns. Fireworks can cause deep burns. Hold burned hands and fingers in cold water. Give pain killers such as ibuprofen (*Advil, Motrin*). Seek medical attention.

- For eye injuries.
  - **DON'T DELAY. SEEK EXPERT MEDICAL ATTENTION IMMEDIATELY.**
  - Don't panic. Stay calm.
  - Don't rub the eye.
  - Don't rinse out the eye.
  - Don't apply any ointment.
  - To prevent a child from rubbing the eye, shield it with the bottom half of a styrofoam cup taped to the brow, bridge of nose, and cheek bone.
  - Don't give ibuprofen or aspirin. These might increase bleeding.

LIGHTNING INJURIES

It is often said that you are more likely to be struck by lightning than win the lottery! Sadly, this may be true. Lightning causes more deaths each year than tornadoes. In some years it has caused more deaths in the United States than any other natural disaster. The good news is that most people who are struck by lightening do **not** die, but many are left with severe injuries.

Lightning occurs most commonly in the summer months, the afternoon being the typical time of the day. Lightning injuries are especially prevalent in mountainous areas and around large bodies of water, such as river basins and lakes. A significant number of injuries occur in persons **who are inside their homes or places of employment!** These injuries are fortunately not likely to be fatal.

One of the most dangerous times for a fatal strike is before a storm! Lightning may travel nearly horizontally as far as ten miles in front of a storm and seem to come out of the clear blue sky when there is still some sunshine! Violent and fast-moving storms are particularly likely to produce lightning. **Lightning strikes may also occur up to thirty minutes after the storm is over!** This has given rise to the **30/30** rule: if there is less than 30 seconds between seeing the lightning and hearing the thunder, you are close enough to be struck. The second 30 is to warn you not to venture out until 30 minutes have passed since the end of the storm.

Lightning may strike you directly but more frequently you will be harmed by a lightning **"splash"** which takes place when lightning that has struck a nearby object such as a tree or fence, **"splashes"** on you. This may happen if you wait out the storm in small shelter such as you may

find on a golf course or on a hiking path. The lightning
strikes the shelter and then splashes on you. This may
also happen if you take shelter under a tall tree. You are
more likely to be struck by lightning directly if you are
out in the open. It is a myth that lightning never strikes
in the same place twice!

Objects that contain metal or that are taller than you,
such as golf clubs or umbrellas, may act as conductors
and significantly increase the chances of a direct lightning strike.

Avoiding lightning injury.

1. Be aware of weather conditions and weather predictions
   before going on excursions, playing sports outside or
   working out in the open. Watch out for darkening skies
   and increasing wind. Remember that lightning may
   strike **before** the storm starts and **after** it is over. **If
   you can hear the thunder, you are probably close
   enough to be struck! Seek shelter.**

2. Tips for finding adequate shelter:
   - Shelter in a substantial building or in an all-metal
     vehicle, such as a car. Roll up the windows and don't
     touch metal surfaces inside or outside the vehicle.
     Lightning can strike automobiles, but the current will
     be conducted by the metal surfaces to the ground.
   - Avoid convertibles and cloth-top jeeps.
   - Do not seek shelter in small sheds, gazebos, or picnic
     or golfing shelters, especially if these are isolated or
     exposed.
   - Stay away from tall trees.
   - Tents offer very little protection and the metal
     support pole actually may act as a lightning rod.

Occupants of a tent should stay away from the poles and from the wet cloth.

- In the forest, seek shelter in a low area amongst smaller trees.

3. If you are unable to find shelter, do not stand near tall, isolated trees, on hilltops, or in exposed areas. If you are totally in the open, stay away from single trees to avoid lightning splashes. **Stay away from metal objects** such as flag poles, motorcycles, tractors, fences, and bicycles. Put down metal objects such as ice picks, axes, hunting knives, umbrellas, and golf clubs

4. **You do not want to be the tallest object around!** Decrease your height by crouching down, kneeling, squatting, or sitting cross-legged on the ground. Do not hold an umbrella above your head and if your backpack projects above you, lay it down.

5. Try to minimize how much of your body comes in contact with the ground. Keep your feet as close together as possible. Do not lie down.

6. Hold your hands over your ears to minimize ear damage from thunderclaps.

7. If you are with a group of people, spread out and stay several yards apart. In the event of a strike, fewer people will be injured by ground currents or by side flashes between people.

8. Avoid swimming, boating, or being the tallest object near a large, open body of water. If you are on the water, head for shore.

9. If indoors during a thunderstorm, avoid being near open doors and windows, fireplaces, metal objects such as pipes, sinks and radiators, and plug-in electrical appliances. Do not use the telephone or the computer. Do not use a cell phone as you can get ear damage from the static.

NOTES:

- Lightning more frequently causes injury than death. If death occurs, it is most likely due to immediate cardiac or cardio-respiratory arrest. Institution of CPR may be lifesaving.

- It is a myth that the lightning victim retains the charge once he or she has been struck. It is totally safe to touch a person who has just been struck by lightning. The sooner you start CPR, the more likely it is to be successful. This is the one time you should attempt to resuscitate the "dead" person first!

- Lightning injuries may cause severe brain damage, burns, eye and ear injuries, and many other types of injuries. **All victims of lightning strikes, even if they appear well, should be taken to the nearest emergency room for assessment.**

DROWNING

Drowning is one of the most common causes of childhood death in the United States. In some states it is *the* leading cause of childhood death! On average, one child drowns every day in a backyard swimming pool. Drowning is also one of the more common causes of death while on vacation.

In the home setting, drowning may occur in the bathtub, the toilet, a bucket, a water barrel, a children's play pool, or the backyard swimming pool. Drowning also frequently happens during water recreational activities such as sailing, canoeing, or swimming in a river, lake, or the sea.

There are two peaks in the age incidence of drowning. The first is the toddler age group where drowning may occur in the bathtub or in as little as one inch of water in a bucket. Water holds an endless fascination for many of us, but especially for children! Young children are naturally inquisitive and seem to be instinctively drawn to water. The second peak in the incidence of drowning is during adolescence and here males predominate. Boys tend to be risk-takers and also seem to be especially lacking in common sense at this age! In older adolescents, alcohol may play a role in drowning incidents.

Prevention of drowning.

Prevention, prevention, prevention! You may be lucky enough to arrive in time to resuscitate your child but this is not the way to prevent death by drowning.

- **Never leave your child alone in the bathtub,** not even to answer the doorbell or the telephone.
- Do not leave buckets of water around.

- Empty your child's play pool once your child has finished swimming.
- Teach your child how to swim at a young age.
- No one should swim alone.
- Swimming pools should be **fenced on all four sides** with a fence that is at least four feet high. The gate should be self-closing and self-latching. Keep a telephone close so that you do not need to leave the pool area to answer it. In the event of an accident the telephone will be close by should you need to call 911.

    I grew up in sunny South Africa in a home with a swimming pool. It did not have a fence around it. (In those days very few pools did.) One day my younger brother went missing. We all raced to the swimming pool to see if he was there. It was mid-winter and we had not bothered to keep the water clean. The water was murky so we all jumped in to look for his body. Fortunately it was not there. We found him later inside asleep behind the sofa, but I still shudder each time I think of the incident!

  — Keep the water clean.
  — If your child goes missing, look in the pool first.
- If you have a swimming pool, learn how to do CPR and keep your certification up to date.
- **Never leave young children alone around water. Responsible adult supervision is the most important aspect in the prevention of drowning.**
- Teach your child safe water behavior.
- Do not allow diving into shallow water.
- When boating, everyone should wear an approved life vest or life jacket which is able to support the wearer so

that the head is above water even if the person is unconscious. A responsible and capable adult should be present during all boating activities.

- Respect the sea! Dangerous back currents and side washes can get the better of even the most powerful swimmer. Swim where there are life guards. Obey their instructions. If they tell you to get out of the water, get out!

- Counsel adolescents about the dangers of drinking and swimming. This is just as bad as drinking and driving!

- Begin CPR immediately if your child is found unconscious in the pool. And call 911.

BREATHING DIFFICULTIES

There are many reasons why an infant or child may have trouble breathing. The causes of breathing difficulty range from a seemingly minor illness such as a stuffy nose (especially in an infant) to more serious causes such as severe asthma and pneumonia. Elsewhere in this book there are discussions on asthma, croup and cough. Refer to these where indicated. Below are guidelines on how to assess if your child is having significant breathing problems and is seriously ill.

1. **The overall appearance of your child and her activity level.** These are very sensitive guides to the severity of childhood illness including the degree of breathing difficulty. Observe your child and ask yourself the following questions.

   - Does she really look ill? Does she appear anxious?
   - What is she doing? Is she playing actively and happily or does she just want to sit quietly on your lap?
   - Does she show any interest in her surroundings?
   - Is she interacting normally with you? Will she make eye contact? Will she smile?

2. **Her breathing pattern.**

   - Is your child breathing in her usual way or **is she struggling to breathe?**
   - Is her breathing smooth and regular? Are there periods of breath holding? Most newborns and babies in the first few months of life have very irregular breathing patterns: They breathe quickly, then slow down, and then hold their breath for ten to fifteen seconds. Just when you are convinced they have totally stopped breathing, they start up again! This breathing pattern is known as "periodic respiration" and is normal at this

age. If an older child has this pattern when asleep one should think of sleep apnea due to enlarged tonsils or adenoids. Deep, sighing respiration may indicate dehydration or out-of-control diabetes.

3. How fast is your child breathing?

Newborn infants often breathe around forty times a minute and at times much faster. After feeding or crying the respiratory rate may get as high as eighty times a minute or faster! After a minute or two, this rapid breathing should settle back to normal. A very good time to count your infant's respirations is when she is asleep. Count the number of breaths over a two minute period and divide the number by two. Older children and adults usually breathe about twenty times a minute. A persistently high respiratory rate (above sixty times a minute in a child less than one year of age or above forty times a minute in an older child) is often an indication that something more serious is happening. This may just be a blocked nose (typically in a young infant), or it may be a sign of a more serious condition such as asthma, bronchiolitis, or pneumonia. Many other diseases such as heart disease or dehydration may also cause your child to breathe rapidly. If your child has a high fever she may also breathe faster than normal.

4. Is she making unusual noises when she breathes?

- If your child has **stridor or croup,** you may hear a high-pitched, harsh sound **as she breathes in.** This is often accompanied by the typical croupy cough which is "barky" and "seal-like". When your child talks you will usually notice hoarseness. Croup often comes on suddenly in the evening.

- Is your child **wheezing?** Wheezing usually is more marked when your child breathes out and is present in many childhood diseases including asthma and bronchiolitis. Bronchiolitis is a viral disease which typically occurs in the winter months in young children.

- A child may generate a variety of strange and disturbing sounds when she breathes through mucus in her nose or throat. These include "snuffling" sounds, wheezing sounds and loose, "junky," "fruity," or "mucousy" coughs. You may think that your child is really ill and are convinced the "mucus is in his chest" but on closer inspection your child is often unperturbed by all the noise and not in any distress!

NOTE: A blocked nose may be a serious problem in a baby. Try blocking your own nose and see how it affects you! If you don't open your mouth you will soon be in serious trouble! Infants don't automatically open their mouths to breathe. Some saline (salt water) down the nose followed by suctioning may cure the problem.

5. Are there any **other signs of respiratory distress?** These include:

- **Retractions,** also known as **recessing.** Each time your child breathes you will notice sucking in of the tissues above the collar bones and between and below the ribs. The abdomen may also suck in with each respiration.
- **Flaring.** If your child's nostrils flare in and out (like a horse's) with each respiration, she is said to have flaring.

Flaring and retractions are both signs of significant respiratory distress. They also may be present in dehydration and shock.

- **Color changes.** Does your child look **pale?** Is there a **bluish discoloration** of the lips or fingertips? This is known as "cyanosis." **Cyanosis only develops late in respiratory disease and should be taken seriously!** Infants with serious infections may also be pale and cyanosed.

NOTE: At times, young infants have very blue hands and feet. This is usually a sign of poor circulation, which is normal in infants, and seldom indicates any serious underlying disease. Older children who are cold also may have blue lips, hands, and feet. They should "pink up" with warming. These children will appear otherwise well and don't have any other signs of respiratory distress.

6. **Does your child complain of any symptoms?** An older child may complain of chest tightness, difficulty breathing, or chest pain. It is worthwhile to know that **children and adults with longstanding breathing problems such as chronic asthma may not complain of any symptoms despite having severe lung disease!**

(If your child has a cough in addition to breathing difficulties, refer to the section on cough as well, page 235.)

How your child is behaving and acting may be more important than any one individual sign mentioned above. If your child is active and running about, she probably does not have severe pneumonia or breathing difficulties even though she may have noisy breathing and a loud cough. On the other hand, a child who is quiet, inactive, and anxious may be in severe respiratory distress but have no cough or apparent breathing difficulty. **Observe your child closely.**

REASONS TO SEEK MEDICAL CARE

1. Your child appears ill.

2. Your child is struggling to breathe.

3. Your child has cyanosis (bluish discoloration) and this is not just due to poor circulation (see above).

4. Your child's respiratory rate is persistently elevated.

5. Your child has retractions and nasal flaring.

6. Your child is very pale.

7. Your child has severe croup or wheezing.

8. Your child complains of chest tightness or chest pain.

9. Your child has a persistent cough.

10. Your child may have none of the above symptoms or signs but your parental intuition tells you there is something seriously wrong. **If in doubt, seek medical care!**

CHOKING PREVENTION AND FIRST AID FOR CHOKING CHILDREN

As always, prevention should come first! People of any age can choke but children younger than four are particularly prone to choking.

Prevention of choking.

1) Foods that easily lead to choking in young children include peanuts and other nuts, popcorn, hard candy, pieces of hot dog, and raw carrots. Do not give nuts and hard candy to young children. Cut food into small pieces before feeding it to young children.

2) Do not let your child eat while running or playing. Supervise eating and mealtimes.

3) Keep small toys and other small objects away from your children. Select toys appropriate for your child's age. Latex balloons are particularly dangerous, as are eraser tips, buttons and button batteries.

4) Instruct the older children in your house not to give infants and younger children pieces of food or small objects.

5) **Learn CPR.** Take a course at your local hospital, American Red Cross or similar organization. Update and practice your skills frequently. Renew your certification regularly, at least every two years.

First aid for choking.

Most choking episodes in children occur while eating or playing and are often witnessed by adults who can intervene while the child is still conscious and responsive. If your child appears to be choking, the first question to ask yourself is "Should I intervene?"

- Do **not** start first aid for choking if your child can cry or talk, has a strong cough, or is breathing adequately.

- Start first aid for choking if your child cannot cough, talk, or emit normal sounds, is changing color (turning blue or pale), cannot breathe, or an older child indicates the universal sign of choking (hands clutching the neck). If a child is found unconscious, you should always suspect upper airway obstruction as a possible cause and initiate appropriate first aid.

Call 911 after starting rescue efforts.

▶ **Infants less than one year of age.** If your baby appears to be choking, his breathing is obstructed, or he is turning blue and trying to cry but just making weak sounds, you will need to intervene:

    — Lay your baby face down with his head low along your forearm. His legs will straddle your forearm. Give five sharp **back blows** between his shoulder blades.

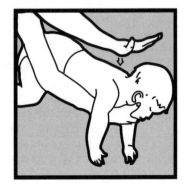

— If this fails to clear the blockage, turn your baby over and give five **chest thrusts** using two fingers on the lower half of the breast bone.

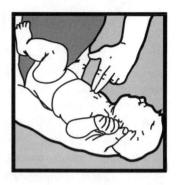

Look in the mouth to see if this has dislodged anything. If the blockage does not clear, call 911. Repeat the above steps until the blockage has cleared or until help arrives. If your child stops breathing or remains blue, start CPR. See point B in this chapter for management of the unconscious infant.

▶ **Older children.**

A) **Conscious child.**

If your child appears to be choking but is coughing, crying, or speaking, encourage your child to cough forcefully and try to expel the foreign body.

If your child cannot breathe or make a sound, then you need to intervene with the Heimlich maneuver. If this does not dislodge the object and she loses consciousness, try abdominal thrusts. If she becomes blue or stops breathing, start CPR. Call 911.

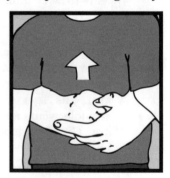

Quick upward thrust just above the navel.

B) Unconscious infant and child.

If you come across an unconscious child, you should always consider a foreign body or upper airway obstruction as a reason for the unconsciousness. This is more likely to be the case if the child is not breathing normally or is blue. Make sure the child is unresponsive. Shout for help. Open the airway and check for breathing. If the victim is not breathing, attempt rescue breathing. If the victim's chest does not rise, reposition the head and try the rescue breathing again. If you still are unable to give effective breaths (the chest does not rise), perform abdominal thrusts in a child or back blows in an infant. After each set of five abdominal thrusts (child) or five back blows (infant), open the victim's mouth to see if you can see a foreign body. If you can see a foreign body, try to hook it out with your finger. If you cannot see a foreign body, do not put a finger in the mouth as it may push an object deeper in. If you do not see a foreign body, repeat the cycle. Call 911. If the victim is not breathing, give rescue breaths until help arrives. Assess pulse/circulation and if necessary begin CPR.

CPR AND BASIC LIFE SUPPORT (BLS)

It is strongly recommended that all parents learn CPR and basic life support. These cannot be learned from books or texts but you should seek out classes in your area. Classes are often provided by your local hospital and by the local chapter of the American Red Cross.

DON'T PUT THIS OFF! Phone today to reserve your place!

Renew your certification at least every two years.

Index

O

oral rehydration solutions. *See* electrolyte solutions
otitis externa (swimmer's ear), 231, 233–234
otitis media, 191, 231–232
ounces, conversion to milliliters, 274

P

pain, 220–222
  abdominal, 279–282
  in ears, 231
  in legs, 221
  eye infection with, 249
  headache, 287–288
  and vomiting, 278
paracetamol, 20
passports, 93–94
pasteurization, 133
Pepto Bismol, 32, 110–112, 122, 271
permethrin, 315, 318–319
pertussis vaccine, 88
pharyngitis, 227
photoconjunctivitis, 311
photokeratitis, 311
photophobia, 249
"pink eye," 245–249
pit vipers, 331
Pneumococcal vaccine, 89
poison ivy/contact dermatitis, 154, 334–338
poison oak, 336
poison sumac, 336
poisoning, 365–369
  prevention, 365–366
  treatment, 366–368
polio vaccine, 88

pounds, conversion to kilograms, 274
pressure immobilization, 332
prickly heat, 148–149
probiotics, 113
projectile vomit, 204, 275, 277
pseudoephedrine nasal decongestant medication, 27–28
pupils (eye), 250

Q

quarts, conversion to liters, 274
quinolone antibiotic, 125

R

rabies, 370, 382–383
raccoons, rabies from, 382
rash, 291–297. *See also* diaper rash; skin problems
  in newborn, 200
  poison ivy/contact dermatitis, 334–338
rattlesnakes, 331
Reye's Syndrome, Pepto Bismol and, 111
rheumatic fever, 228
rifaximin, 125
ringworm, 153–154, 190
risks in travel, children vs. adults, 80–81
Rocky Mountain spotted fever, 321
rubella vaccine, 88
"runny nose," 223–226

S

saline nose drops, 28–29, 202, 224, 243–244
salmon patches, 200
salt water, 28–29

428 PEDIATRIC TRAVEL BOOK